The transmission of health practices (c. 1500 to 2000)

Medizin,
Gesellschaft und Geschichte

Jahrbuch
des Instituts für Geschichte der Medizin
der Robert Bosch Stiftung

herausgegeben von
Robert Jütte

Beiheft 39

The transmission of health practices (c. 1500 to 2000)

edited by Martin Dinges and Robert Jütte

Franz Steiner Verlag Stuttgart
2011

Umschlagabbildung: Krankenpflegekurs des Vereins für Homöo-
pathie und Lebenspflege 1886 e. V. Heidenheim im Schwanen-
keller; 1926

© Bildarchiv des Instituts für Geschichte der Medizin der Robert
Bosch Stiftung

Gedruckt mit freundlicher Unterstützung der Robert Bosch
Stiftung GmbH

Bibliografische Information der Deutschen Nationalbibliothek:
Die Deutsche Nationalbibliothek verzeichnet diese
Publikation in der Deutschen Nationalbibliografie;
detaillierte bibliografische Daten sind im Internet über
<http://dnb.d-nb.de> abrufbar.

ISBN 978-3-515-09897-7

Contents

Introduction

Martin Dinges and Robert Jütte

Although the social history of medicine[1] has developed rapidly over the last two decades and covers a plethora of issues, little attention has been paid to understanding the transmission of health knowledge from the different health agents to the various target groups[2]. Health knowledge, while not sufficient to modify health behaviour, is a necessary component of behavioural change. Knowledge areas include chronic disease, communicable disease, consumer health, environmental health, human sexuality, mental health, nutrition, physical fitness, and drug use/abuse.

The bulk of medico-historical research in this area concentrates on the educational campaigns organized and carried out by professional health agents, both medical and non-medical, for example physicians[3] and teachers[4]. Both professional groups are trained and convinced that they represent the contact point with the community and that they are the means for the transmission of health knowledge and of information for mothers and children as well as for the community in general. But whether their educational programmes and campaigns really led to changes in health behaviour, is hardly known. Self reports such as diaries, memoirs and other autobiographical documents, could be sources for historical research on this subject. A survey of recent health education programmes designed to reduce health risks and control costs shows that the 32 programmes included in this study led to an average reduction of 20 per cent in health benefit claims.[5]

What is even more important is that not only physicians and teachers are involved in promoting health but also other professions such as social workers and nurses. We know little about their efforts and achievements in transmitting medical advice. Also hardly anything is known of how intergenerational transmission of health knowledge and behaviour worked in the past.[6] An interesting question in this context is how health knowledge is transmitted over generations. Are the traditional mechanisms still intact that have been in place in the past? These are complex questions and they require detailed historical

---

1   Faure (1990); Dinges: Social History (2004); Eckart/Jütte (2007), pp. 156 ff.
2   For the reproduction and dissemination of health knowledge from a medical sociological point of view, see Dingwall/Heath/Reid/Stacy (1977); Bourdelais/Faure (2005); Faure (1999).
3   Loetz (1990); Ischreyt (1990).
4   Krei (1995); Henner (1998); Pfefferkorn (2002); Noel (1999).
5   Fries/Koop/Sokolov/Beadle/Wright (1998).
6   For a case study based on letters exchanged among pietists in early modern Württemberg, see Ernst (2003). For the 19th and 20th century, cf. McCray Beier (2009). For a modern study, see, for instance, Hafetz (2006); Al-Ansari/Honkala/Honkala (2003).

evidence, which is extremely elusive and difficult to unearth from the archives. There is also a need to explore the role of men within the family and gender specific health practices.[7]

The biennial Anglo-Dutch-German Workshop, a cooperation between the Institute for the History of Medicine of the Robert Bosch Foundation (Stuttgart), the Wellcome Trust Centre for the History of Medicine (London), the Centre of the History of Medicine (Warwick) and the Medical Centre University (Utrecht), which was held at the Institute for the History of Medicine of the Robert Bosch Foundation in 2009, therefore focused on strategies for the transmission of medical knowledge from early modern times to the present. The health practices selected for discussion in this workshop were, among others, maternity and pregnancy, prevention of venereal diseases, dental hygiene, drug addiction and alcohol abuse, nursing skills and techniques, childcare, and mental health. One of the reasons for this selection was that most of these practices have not yet been studied from the transmitter's point of view, but rather from a more general perspective.[8] Other interesting and important topics not included here are, for example, lay groups supporting alternative therapies[9] and the 'lay, non-professional, non-specialist, popular culture arena in which illness is first defined and health care activities initiated'[10] (Arthur Kleinman). Given the fact that there has already been considerable analysis of the role of physicians in the transmission of health knowledge, the workshop focused on other health agents, while keeping in mind that health practices develop from a complex interplay of factors, including income, education, gender, age, social support, cultural background and physical environment, which create a range of life contexts within which an individual's capacity to adopt healthy practices is either enhanced or restrained.

The participants in this workshop who came from Britain, Holland, Germany, Austria and Switzerland discussed ways in which health practices were transmitted and how they affected the health strategies within the population. All contributors were asked to put an emphasis on the ways in which people in the past were exposed to health care knowledge. As expected it proved difficult to find out whether the transmission of health knowledge changed the health practices of people, paying special attention to the acquirement of skills and knowledge. In addition to this we wanted to identify a range of issues and barriers relating to the acquisition of medical knowledge in specific health care settings. Consideration was also given to the gap between the rhetoric of

---

7   Dinges: Mütter und Söhne (2004); Schweig (2009).
8   For relevant literature on some of these topics, see, for example, Marks (1994); Bock/ Thane (1991); Stokes (2003); Daalen/Gijswijt-Hofstra (1998); Sauerteig (1999); Sauerteig/ Davidson (2009); Türp (1990); Crowley (1999); Murdock (2002); Hey/Rickling/Stockhecke/Thau (2004); Hauschildt (1995); Buhler-Wilkerson (2001); Rafferty (1996); Hähner-Rombach (2009); Warren (2006); Dill (1997); Stöckel (1996); Usborne (1995).
9   Dinges: Medizinkritische Bewegungen (1996); Regin (1995).
10 Kleinman (1980), p. 50. For a historical study of this part of the health care system, see Jütte (1991).

the values underpinning health policies, and the practice and provision of health care. The role played by family and social milieu in the transmission of health practices was explored. A further point of interest was the patient response to new health care concepts and the formation of patient networks. The knowledge transmission to Catholic and Protestant sisterhoods, the conveyance of knowledge to wet nurses, the role of clergymen as conveyers of medical knowledge and, lastly, the transmission practices of health authorities and private charities were also under consideration.

The present volume includes selected papers from this workshop. The original division into five categories has been retained: The articles which have been chosen and revised for publication deal with the following 'transmitters':

1. Family and kin
2. Patients and self-help organizations
3. Nurses
4. Social workers and health officers
5. Clergy and religious institutions

There can be no doubt that the theme of the transmission and implementation of medical knowledge holds great potential for the future research of the history of medicine whose scientific discourse can be fruitfully enhanced by the categories of practice exploration. However, the concept of 'transmission' and pertaining problems need more attention. Some of the aspects which could not be addressed in this volume are the transmission of practices of hygiene and health concepts among soldiers.[11] It also has to be mentioned in this context that we still do not know much about the long term effects of military service on the change of health practices. The prevention of venereal diseases due to health education during military service could also be an interesting case study in this respect.

Family and kin

Mothers have been and still are important gatekeepers in the health care system. *Angela Davis (Coventry)* looks into the situation of women experiencing maternity in Great Britain after 1945. She shows how women acquired knowledge of pregnancy, childbirth and infant care. While it was mostly the family, particularly the mother, who advised the pregnant woman before 1945, physicians, health authorities and the media offered extensive advice and care programmes after World War II. Contradicting the prevailing assumption that mothers, friends and relatives played less and less of a role in the knowledge transmission process on childbirth and infant care, Davis, who based her ana-

---

11   Dinges: Soldatenkörper (1996).

lysis on 165 interviews with women in Oxfordshire and Berkshire, demonstrated that knowledge transmission remained widely within lay circles and that the social surroundings continued to act as an important source of advice.

Willemijn Ruberg (Utrecht) explored the question of who, in nineteenth century Holland, had the expertise to determine whether a woman had been raped and how this might affect her health. She argued that it was mostly the mothers who became aware of changes in their daughters' bodies and who noticed the first signs of venereal disease. They were the first to examine the young rape victims and take them to the doctor. Sometimes it was they who treated their daughters. Ruberg pointed out that the history of medicine has so far not considered the role of the mothers whose knowledge, on the treatment of venereal disease for instance, was based on experience. She also showed that physicians, midwives, pharmacists and mothers interpreted the signs of rape in different ways.

Susanne Hoffmann (Stuttgart) based her contribution on the observation that, around 1900, traditional dental care was replaced by the new preventive dental hygiene. She investigates how the new approach was implemented within the population. Among the lower classes and in rural areas the transformation lasted until the middle of the twentieth century. Hoffmann's research which she based principally on the evaluation of 155 autobiographies indicates that children were the driving force behind the change as they carried the new hygiene practices into their families. It is assumed that they acquired their knowledge at school where dentists promoted their dental health care programmes. The marketing strategies of the dental industry probably also played a part.

Patients and self-help organizations

Gemma Blok (Amsterdam) chose the treatment of addiction as a case study for the role of self-help groups as mediators in the health care system. She analyses the 'Medical and Social Service for Heroin Users' (Medisch-sociale Dienst voor Heroïne Gebruikers) which was founded in 1977 and the Rotterdam Junkie Union (founded in 1980). During this time Holland was in the grip of a 'heroin epidemic'. The aim of both organizations was to reduce drug consumption rather than try to achieve total abstinence, to 'care' instead of 'cure'. They wanted to integrate drug users back into society, to support and treat them like 'normal' persons. The junkie organizations supported 'alternative' forms of addiction treatment like walk-in shelters and consumption rooms, and wanted to liberate drug users from both the justice system, and the pressure of the drug user scene.

Nurses

Nurses were among the most important groups transmitting health practices. *Carmen M. Mangion (Manchester)* studies the acquisition of knowledge by the Catholic religious women in nineteenth-century Britain. Only few of the nursing sisters had received formal medical training as the church law of the time did not allow that. As a consequence the nursing sisters founded informal, local and international, 'knowledge networks' where knowledge was passed on from sister to sister or from physician to sister. Their lack of formal training meant that they were dependent on the physicians. Most important was the pastoral care that they carried out independently of the physician.

Karen Nolte (Würzburg) looks into the parish work of the deaconesses. Rooted as he was in traditional Protestantism the German pastor Theodor Fliedner (1800–1864) who opened the first deaconesses' hospital near Düsseldorf, saw a connection between sickness, poverty and faithlessness and he tried to find access to the souls of the poor by caring for the sick. Evaluation of the letters that the deaconesses wrote to Fliedner and his wife gives insight into the deaconesses' everyday life among the poor. Karen Nolte demonstrated which transmission mechanisms were applied by the deaconesses in order to pass on their medical knowledge and alleviate the material needs. Her sources also show to which extent their care for the soul was valued. As poverty and sickness were seen as the consequence of an alienation from God, it was the sisters' task to go to the families and unearth the source of corruption. The deaconesses succeeded in establishing their own area of competence that was independent of the physicians.

Social workers and health officers

Andreas Weigl (Vienna) describes the rise and 'fall' of female health care workers in Austria in the early twentieth century. Because of the high mortality rate of infants the government had made special health care workers available. It was their expressed aim to improve the health situation of children and adolescents. As part of their tasks they had to educate the mothers and teach them to fulfil their tasks and duties. They also advised them on hygiene and nursing. Health care workers were also sent to combat tuberculosis. During National Socialism the health care worker was replaced by the 'people's welfare worker' (*Volkspflegerin*) who had merely a control and executive function and could come dangerously close to the Nazi elimination ideology. After World War II, it was – next to the loss of prestige due to the Nazi regime – the futher drop in infant mortality that led to the fast reduction in the number of these health care workers. They were replaced in the 1970s by social workers.

John Stewart's (Glasgow) topic is 'British Child Guidance' where professional and lay knowledge came together. This organization was a medical-psychiatric initiative that had been established after World War I, first in the

United States and then also in Great Britain and Europe. The basic premise of this organization was that each child, no matter how normal he or she might appear on the outside, experienced maladjustment at one stage or another in his or her life. If the problem was not recognized it could lead to further problems in later life. The fact that the young patients would encounter representatives of three professional groups, psychiatrists, psychologists and (psychiatric) social workers, turned out to be problematic: the leading figure was the psychiatrist who was responsible for diagnosis and treatment. But the members of the psychiatric social service, who were always women, had the closer contact. They gathered the material on which the suggested treatment would be based. Although they had some theoretical basic knowledge of psychiatry this still meant that diagnoses and prognoses were ultimately determined by medically unqualified staff.

Clergy and religious institutions

Andreas Golob (Graz) provides an example of how priests made use of popular media for health education in the later enlightenment era. From the repertoire of sources he draws on, Johann Jakob Gabriel, a Catholic priest and catechist, stands out with his Socratic stories, a very early example of a collection entirely devoted to health issues. Contextualization was achieved mostly through the description of pastoral tasks within the health care system during the Habsburg monarchy around 1800. Apart from administering the sacraments, primarily the anointing of the sick, enlightened priests advocated additional, mostly preventive, measures for health maintenance and the consultation of registered health advisers. They tried to reach broad parts of the population through personal contact, sermons, Sunday school and religion lessons. The stories give insight into the transmission of culture and knowledge from authors from the states of Prussia and Saxony. The analysis centres on physical, psychological, social and religious aspects of health and sickness.

    That religious institutions still play a role in transmitting health practices is shown by *Harry Oosterhuis (Maastricht)* who describes the change in attitude towards homosexuality that occurred in the Catholic communities in Holland in the 1950s and 1960s. He documents how the discourse among the medical profession influenced the views of the Catholic clergy. A dialogue conducted among priests, physicians, psychiatrists, psychologists and Catholic homosexuals led to the social and psychological re-evaluation of homosexuality which had so far been regarded as sinful and pathological. Priests and Catholic psychiatrists began to support Catholic homosexuals by helping them to find a lifestyle that was compatible with religious values. The priests' attitude remained ambivalent, as their behaviour was moralizing on the one hand, while they counselled homosexuals like social workers and psychotherapists on the other. It seems that pastoral care for homosexuals was developed further and consolidated. The medical view did, however, not replace that of the clergymen.

Bibliography

Al-Ansari, Jassem; Honkala, Eino; Honkala, Sisko: Oral health knowledge and behavior among male health sciences college students in Kuwait. In: BMC Oral Health 3 (2003), no. 2, pp. 1–6.

Bock, Gisela; Thane, Pat (eds.): Maternity and gender policies: Women and the rise of the European welfare states, 1880s-1950s. London et al 1991.

Bourdelais, Patrice; Faure, Olivier (eds.): Les nouvelles pratiques de santé: acteurs, objets, logiques sociales (XVIIIe-XXe siècles). Paris 2005.

Buhler-Wilkerson, Karen: No place like home: a history of nursing and home care in the United States. Baltimore 2001.

Crowley, John W. (ed.): Drunkard's progress: narratives of addiction, despair, and recovery. Baltimore 1999.

Daalen, Rineke van; Gijswijt-Hofstra, Marijke (eds.): Gezond en wel: vrouwen en de zorg voor gezondheid in de twintigste eeuw. Amsterdam 1998.

Dill, Gregor: Nationalsozialistische Säuglingspflege und Kleinkinderpädagogik: eine frühe Erziehung zum Massenmenschen. Lizentiatsarbeit Univ. Bern 1997.

Dinges, Martin (ed.): Medizinkritische Bewegungen im Deutschen Reich (ca. 1870-ca. 1933). Stuttgart 1996.

Dinges, Martin: Soldatenkörper in der Frühen Neuzeit. Erfahrungen mit einem unzureichend geschützten, formierten und verletzten Körper in Selbstzeugnissen. In: Dülmen, Richard van (ed.): KörperGeschichten. Studien zur historischen Kulturforschung. Frankfurt/Main 1996, pp. 71–98.

Dinges, Martin: Mütter und Söhne (ca. 1450-ca. 1850): Ein Versuch anhand von Briefen. In: Flemming, Jens; Puppel, Pauline (eds.): Lesarten der Geschichte: Ländliche Ordnungen und Geschlechterverhältnisse. Festschrift für Heide Wunder zum 65. Geburtstag. Kassel 2004, pp. 89–119.

Dinges, Martin: Social History of Medicine in Germany and France in the Late Twentieth Century: From the History of Medicine toward a History of Health. In: Huisman, Frank; Warner, John Harley (eds.): Locating Medical History: The Stories and their Meanings. Baltimore 2004, pp. 209–236.

Dingwall, Robert; Heath, Christian; Reid, Margaret; Stacy, Margaret (eds.): Health Care and Health Knowledge. London 1977.

Eckart, Wolfgang U.; Jütte, Robert: Medizingeschichte. Eine Einführung. Köln 2007.

Ernst, Katharina: Die medikale Kultur württembergischer Pietisten im 18. Jahrhundert. Stuttgart 2003.

Faure, Olivier: The social history of health in France: a survey of recent developments. In: Social History of Medicine 3 (1990), pp. 437–445.

Faure, Olivier (ed.): Les thérapeutiques: savoirs et usages. Annecy 1999.

Fries, James F.; Koop, C. Everett; Sokolov, Jacque; Beadle, Carson E.; Wright, Daniel: Beyond Health Promotion: Reducing Need and Demand for Medical Care. In: Health Affairs 17 (1998), pp. 70–84.

Hähner-Rombach, Sylvelyn (ed.): Alltag in der Krankenpflege: Geschichte und Gegenwart. Stuttgart 2009.

Hafetz, Jessica S.: The intergenerational transmission of health knowledge and behaviors: An evaluation of the Go! Kids Obesity Prevention Program (January 1, 2006). ETD Collection for Fordham University. Paper AAI3255044 (http://fordham.bepress.com/dissertations/AAI3255044).

Hauschildt, Elke: "Auf den richtigen Weg zwingen ...". Trinkerfürsorge 1922 bis 1945. Freiburg/Brsg. 1995.

Henner, Günter: Quellen zur Geschichte der Gesundheitspädagogik: 2500 Jahre Gesundheitsförderung in Texten und Bildern; ein wissenschaftliches Lesebuch. Würzburg 1998.

Hey, Bernd; Rickling, Matthias; Stockhecke, Kerstin; Thau, Bärbel: Alkohol – Sünde oder Sucht? Enthaltsamkeitsbewegung, Trinkerfürsorge und Suchtberatung im evangelischen Westfalen. Bielefeld 2004.

Ischreyt, Irene: Der Arzt als Lehrer: populärmedizinische Publizistik in Liv-, Est- und Kurland als Beitrag zur volkstümlichen Aufklärung im 18. Jahrhundert. Lüneburg 1990.

Jütte, Robert: Ärzte, Heiler und Patienten. Medizinischer Alltag in der frühen Neuzeit. München. Zürich 1991.

Kleinman, Arthur: Patients and Healers in the Context of Culture: An Exploration of the Borderland Between Anthropology Medicine and Psychiatry. Berkeley 1980.

Krei, Thomas: Gesundheit und Hygiene in der Lehrerbildung: Strukturen und Prozesse im Rheinland seit 1870. Köln; Weimar; Wien 1995.

Loetz, Francisca: Leserbriefe als Medium ärztlicher Aufklärungsbemühungen: Johann August Unzers "Der Arzt. Eine medicinische Wochenschrift" als Beispiel. In: Jahrbuch des Instituts für Geschichte der Medizin der Robert Bosch Stiftung 7 (1990), pp. 189–204.

Marks, Lara V.: Model mothers: Jewish mothers and maternity provision in East London 1870–1939. Oxford 1994.

McCray Beier, Lucinda: Health culture in the heartland, 1880–1980: an oral history. Urbana 2009.

Murdock, Catherine Gilbert: Domesticating drink: women, men, and alcohol in America, 1870–1940. Baltimore 2002.

Noel, Rebecca R.: Schooling the body: the intersection of educational and medical reform in New England, 1800–1860. Doctoral thesis, Boston University 1999.

Pfefferkorn, Laura Bigger: School health education in South Carolina 1894–1989: tinkering toward professionalization. Doctoral thesis, University of South Carolina 2002.

Rafferty, Anne-Marie: The politics of nursing knowledge. London et al 1996.

Regin, Cornelia: Selbsthilfe und Gesundheitspolitik: die Naturheilbewegung im Kaiserreich (1889 bis 1914). Stuttgart 1995.

Sauerteig, Lutz: Krankheit, Sexualität, Gesellschaft: Geschlechtskrankheiten und Gesundheitspolitik in Deutschland im 19. und 20. Jahrhundert. Stuttgart 1999.

Sauerteig, Lutz; Davidson, Roger (eds.): Shaping sexual knowledge: a cultural history of sex education in twentieth century Europe. London; New York 2009.

Schweig, Nicole: Gesundheitsverhalten von Männern: Gesundheit und Krankheit in Briefen 1800–1950. Stuttgart 2009.

Stöckel, Sigrid: Säuglingsfürsorge zwischen sozialer Hygiene und Eugenik: das Beispiel Berlins im Kaiserreich und in der Weimarer Republik. Berlin; New York 1996.

Stokes, Patricia R.: Contested conceptions: experiences and discourses of pregnancy and childbirth in Germany, 1914–1933. Ann Arbor 2003.

Türp, Jens C.: Zahnfegen, Zahnpinsel, Zahnputzhölzer: zur Aktualität traditioneller Formen der Mund- und Zahnhygiene. In: Curare 13 (1990), pp. 75–87.

Usborne, Cornelie: The politics of the body in Weimar Germany: women's reproductive rights and duties. 4th ed. Ann Arbor 1995.

Warren, Mame: Our shared legacy: nursing education at Johns Hopkins, 1889–2006. Baltimore 2006.

'When I was young you just went and asked your mother.' The changing role of friends and kin in the transmission of knowledge about maternity in post-1945 Britain[1]

Angela Davis

Introduction

Over the course of the twentieth century infant and maternal mortality rates fell considerably in Britain. Much credit for this improvement has been attributed to the health services and the increasing role of the medical profession in the spheres of childbirth, antenatal and postnatal care and infant welfare. It has generally been accepted that allied to this medicalisation was a transformation in the transmission of knowledge about maternity, with women increasingly reliant on the advice of medical professionals rather than that from traditional sources, such as mothers, friends and kin. While infant welfare clinics and health visitors were the key promoters of modern methods in motherhood, women were exposed to changing ideas from a variety of sources. There were advice columns in national and local newspapers and women's magazines; advertising hoardings urged patent products to safeguard children's health; and health programmes were broadcast on the radio and later television.[2] Coupled to this proliferation of information available to women, increased geographical mobility meant that women often no longer had kin at close hand and therefore needed to obtain their knowledge from other sources. 'Modern' mothers of the post-1945 period have therefore been viewed as keen to reject the 'old wives' tales' of the previous generations seeking out the 'scientific' advice of medical professionals.

In this paper, however, I would like to argue that while it may have been commonly assumed that by the post-war period women dismissed the advice of their mothers, friends and other kin as 'old wives tales' and instead preferred to seek the advice of their doctor, in practice this was not always the case. Based on the results of 165 oral history interviews with Oxfordshire women about their experiences of motherhood in post-1945 Britain I will demonstrate that in reality the transmission of knowledge about maternity through lay sources remained. By analysing the accounts of mothers themselves their continued reliance on the advice of both friends and kin will be revealed. In addition I will demonstrate that when women did reject the advice of their mothers, it was not simply due to their preference for bio-medicine. Issues of generational conflict were also at play. Finally, I will show that

1 This paper draws on research conducted during a Leverhulme Early Career Fellowship. I am grateful to the Trust for their generous support.
2 Peretz (1992), pp. 257–262.

even when they did turn to orthodox medicine, they could still value the practical experience of the caregiver over their professional expertise.

Methodology

The paper is based on oral history interviews with 165 women that were undertaken by the author as part of wider research on women's experiences of motherhood between 1945 and 1990.[3] The women selected were living in different locations in Oxfordshire and Berkshire – rural, urban and suburban. These are the villages of Benson and Ewelme in south Oxfordshire; the Wychwood villages in west Oxfordshire; the twenty-four square miles near Banbury in north Oxfordshire covered by the "Country Planning" (1944) survey[4]; Oxford city centre; the contrasting suburbs of Cowley and Florence Park in east Oxford and North Oxford and Summertown in north Oxford; and the villages of Crowthorne and Sandhurst in Berkshire[5]. The women all lived in Oxfordshire or Berkshire when their children were growing up, but the range of communities they lived in was specifically chosen to enable a comparison of local experiences. As many women as logistically possible were interviewed. While the numbers are significantly lower than for social survey and sampling methods, as Kate Fisher has argued, 'Oral history provides the historian with dense and rich qualitative material rather than strength in numbers.'[6] Interviewees were principally found through community groups, social clubs and by women recommending other women to me. Kate Field believes this 'snowballing', where each respondent gives the name of another person to participate, is a particularly appropriate method for finding respondents to a local study because it helps secure the trust of interviewees through being 'recommended' to them by their friends.[7]

The sample was self-selecting in that all the women had volunteered to be interviewed. However the aim was to construct a sample that ranged in age from their forties to their nineties and represented both middle and working classes[8] and a variety of educational backgrounds (from minimum-age school

---

3   The research has arisen from my DPhil, Davis (2007), and Leverhulme Trust-funded project "Motherhood c. 1970–1990: An Oral History".
4   The Agricultural Economics Research Institute Oxford (1944).
5   The two villages of Sandhurst and Crowthorne in Berkshire were selected in order to complement the Oxfordshire locations thus enabling a comparison between health and welfare provision in the two counties.
6   Fisher (1997), p. 40.
7   Field (2001), p. 103.
8   Interviewees were asked to give their class of origin. Joanna Bourke suggests that this subjective perception of class position 'provides one way around the thorny problem of gender'. She stresses that employing categories such as occupation, income, or relationship to the means of production as indicators of 'class' is clearly problematical when focusing on women. Employed women may be categorised in terms of their own occupation, or that of the 'chief breadwinner' in the household, and women without paid em-

leavers to graduates) to see how locality, education and class influenced women's experiences. The interviews were semi-structured, following the model described by Penny Summerfield[9], and were typically between one and two hours long. However when silences, literal and figurative, were encountered in the narratives time was always given to respondents to allow them to decide how they wished to proceed. To address some of the ethical issues surrounding oral history all the potential respondents were informed in advance of the interview about the aims of the research. They therefore had the opportunity to make decisions about what they would choose to divulge prior to the interview which placed them in a more powerful position.[10] This advance notification also prevented any difference in expectation between interviewer and interviewee. All interviewees were asked to sign copyright and consent forms at the end of the interview whereby they had the chance to specify any restrictions they wished to make on their contributions. Pseudonyms have been used.

Maternal care in Oxfordshire

During the middle decades of the century Oxfordshire was often at the forefront of developments in maternal care. These changes came in part from a forward-looking medical profession, encouraged by the presence of a teaching hospital – there was the early provision of a family planning clinic in 1935 and a move to attaching health visitors to doctors' practices in 1955 – but also because the city attracted influential middle-class intellectuals such as the birth educator Sheila Kitzinger. In both Oxfordshire and the city of Oxford maternal mortality, infant mortality and perinatal mortality rates were generally below the national average. The rates for Oxford also tended to be lower than those for Oxfordshire. There were many significant differences in the maternity care women received from the Oxford Public Health Department and the Oxfordshire Public Health Department, such as in the provision of antenatal classes, child welfare clinics, and the proportion of home-births.[11]

---

ployment are often allocated to the 'class' position of their husband or father. Carolyn Steedman goes further, concluding women are 'without class, because the cut and fall of a skirt and good leather shoes can take you across the river on to the other side: the fairy-tales tell you that goose-girls may marry kings'. However while there clearly are difficulties in defining women by class, the language of class was dominant in the post-war decades, it was clearly influential upon the interviewees' lives and is a useful analytical tool. Bourke (1994), p. 4; Steedman (1986), pp. 15–16.

9   Summerfield (1998), pp. 1–42.
10   Field (2001), pp. 104–105.
11   City of Oxford: Annual Reports of the Medical Officer of Health (hereafter MOH Oxford City); Oxfordshire County Council: Annual Reports of the the County Medical Officer of Health and Principal School Medical Officer (hereafter MOH Oxfordshire); Parfit (1987).

There is an interesting comparison to be made between the two authorities in the provision of care in urban and rural areas. By the 1940s most country women, like their urban counterparts, were attended by the District Nurse, or midwife, although if their doctors prescribed hospital treatment, they went to the Maternity Department at the County Infirmary.[12] However while in the city of Oxford antenatal clinics were available in the 1930s, these were not on offer in rural areas until the late 1960s.[13] In terms of antenatal education Oxfordshire also lagged behind the city. Antenatal classes were not started in Oxfordshire until 1961, and then only two classes were in operation.[14] In Oxford city mothercraft classes were on offer by 1947.[15] Perhaps the most striking difference was in the provision of Family Planning Advice, which showed how far advanced Oxford city was in comparison to Oxfordshire. In the city of Oxford a birth control clinic was started in May 1935 by the Assistant Medical Officer of Health, Dr Mary Fisher, to give birth control advice on medical grounds.[16] With regard to the county, however, the Medical Officer of Health (MOH) did not even mention Family Planning in his report until 1964 and it was not until the Family Planning Act 1967 came into force that the first clinic was set up in the county.[17] The comparison with Reading in Berkshire is also striking. Reading council only set up its first family planning clinic in 1966 with the term 'family planning' banned until 1961.[18]

The numbers of home-births in the city of Oxford were higher than in the county throughout the period. This was principally because the poor living conditions that still existed in rural areas, with houses without electricity and running water, meant that more women were recommended hospital births on social grounds. In 1954, for example, twenty-seven percent of births took place at home in the county, thirty-four percent in Oxford.[19] By the end of the period this difference had levelled off, particularly after the opening of the Churchill's General Practitioner (GP) unit in 1966 which increased the number of beds open to women in Oxford[20] and the policy of discharging home early patients delivered in consultant units was introduced in Oxfordshire to provide for as many hospital births as possible.[21] This rapid move to hospital deliveries throughout Oxfordshire was the result of changes in policy at the national level with local health departments reacting to these pronouncements. The Cranbrook report in 1959 called for seventy percent of births to take

12 The Agricultural Economics Research Institute Oxford (1944), p. 177.
13 MOH Oxford City (1935), p. 84; MOH Oxfordshire (1967), p. 23.
14 MOH Oxfordshire (1961), p. 9.
15 MOH Oxford City (1947), p. 23.
16 MOH Oxford City (1935), p. 84.
17 MOH Oxfordshire (1964), p. 10; MOH Oxfordshire (1967), p. 33.
18 Parfit (1987), p. 95.
19 MOH Oxford City (1954), p. 8; MOH Oxfordshire (1954), p. 19. By the early 1960s the number of home-births in Oxfordshire was further reduced because of a shortage of midwives.
20 MOH Oxford City (1966), p. 10.
21 MOH Oxfordshire (1966), p. 19.

place in hospital.[22] Then in 1970 the Peel Committee recommended provision for 100 percent of confinements to take place in hospital.[23] These national debates and developments were reflected in the care on offer to women in Oxfordshire. In Oxford between 1948 and 1952 between fifty-six percent and sixty percent of deliveries took place in hospital but by 1971 this was ninety-four percent.[24]

Before the creation of the National Health Service (NHS) in 1948 the cost of seeing a doctor meant that access to orthodox health care was beyond the reach of many Oxfordshire residents. Jessica who worked as a GP in Bloxham in north Oxfordshire both before and after the launch of the NHS articulated the change. Asked how it affected the care she was able to provide she told the story of a mother of a sick child. Jessica had enquired from the mother why she had not been called and was told, '"Well my heart sinks when you walk through the gate doctor because I know that's three and sixpence and I can't really afford it", well that was an awful thing [...] and all that was gone with the NHS.'[25] Another GP who qualified in 1947 and practiced in Cowley in Oxford explained how the introduction of the NHS brought

> a great pent up wave [...] people who could begrudge paying money for their children's ailments turning up in their droves in the surgery. You suddenly realised there was a lot more of illness about of a minor or even major nature than was hitherto thought. So there was a great rush of use of the health service in the first few years. But [after that] you didn't see children with neglected fingers looking like a sausage full of puss because parents would bring the child along earlier.[26]

Prior to the introduction of the NHS those people who could not afford to see the doctor therefore sought other means of treating ill-health. Lucinda Beier has demonstrated the centrality of neighbourhood health authorities in Lancashire in the first half of the twentieth century. The main skill of these informal health authorities was their ability to offer diagnoses and advice – whether it involved administering a remedy or consulting someone else, such as a physician or a chemist.[27] People also relied on traditional cures passed down through families. In Oxfordshire, such remedies were particularly adopted by those from working-class and rural backgrounds who had the least access to formal healthcare. For example, recalling her childhood in the village of Adderbury in north Oxfordshire in the 1920s and 1930s Theresa said, 'I remember once when I had a very bad ear, my Dad saying, "Try a drop of olive oil, try the middle out of a boiled walnut, coz the doctor will charge half a crown".' Theresa went on to explain that: 'It turned out I had an abscess in my ear, which all these things happened after measles, and that's why I lost most of

22   Ministry of Health (1959).
23   Department of Health and Social Security (1970).
24   MOH Oxford City (1952), p. 4; MOH Oxford City (1971), p. 87.
25   Jessica, BA8, pp. 7–8.
26   Tait/Graham-Jones (1998), p. 230.
27   Beier (2008), p. 59.

my hearing, and he was a bit sorry after.'[28] This limited access to health care was also seen in relation to maternity services. While the 1902 Midwives Act had limited their ability to practice, village handywomen, who acted as midwives and layers out of the dead, remained important figures into the interwar years when outlawed by the 1936 Midwives Act.[29]

However, running alongside this reliance on traditional forms of health care, was the increasing use of the formal sector. Ann Hardy has noted how working people's access to orthodox medicine was greatly improved during the course of the nineteenth century by the emergence of the insurance principle in the form of friendly societies.[30] This trend continued into the twentieth century and in 1911 Lloyd George introduced a national insurance scheme to fund welfare benefits. However access to this official health care was gendered. Margery Spring Rice revealed the ill-health and inadequate medical care that was still common for working-class women in the 1930s.[31] As Helen Jones has argued, women gained least from the pre-war insurance schemes and were probably hardest hit by poverty during the interwar years.[32] Class and gender also circumscribed doctor-patient encounters.[33] In her 1960s study of general practice Ann Cartwright found that women (of reproductive age) visited their GP more frequently than men, both in their own right and through consulting the doctor about their children. There were also differences in their attitudes towards their doctors. Women attached greater importance to having a doctor who was approachable and listened to them whereas men appreciated 'straightforwardness' and more often mentioned some aspect of his medical care. When asked whether they would discuss a personal problem with their doctor a third of the women thought they might, compared with a quarter of men.[34] Explanations for these gender differences have suggested they result from gendered attitudes to ill-health resulting from the division of labour inside and outside the home,[35] or that it may be more socially acceptable for women to report symptoms and feelings to health professionals.[36] In addition men and women also turn to their GP with different complaints. Factors related to psychological distress seem to be more important to women and physical symptoms to men.[37]

28 Theresa, BA10, p. 16.
29 Donnison (1977), p. 191.
30 Hardy (2001), p. 17.
31 Rice (1939).
32 Jones (1994), pp. 123–124.
33 Digby (1999), pp. 232–233.
34 Cartwright (1967), pp. 186–194. Moreover, these differences have remained. See: Cartwright/Anderson (1981), pp. 157–165; Campbell/Roland (1996); Carr-Hill/Rice/Roland (1996); Scaife/Gill/Heywood/Neal (2000).
35 Cornwell (1984), pp. 139–140.
36 Verbrugge (1989); Möller-Leimkuhler (2002).
37 Kapur/Hunt/Lunt/McBeth/Creed/Macfarlane (2005).

The advice of kin

Women have been held to be central in preserving the unity and coherence of traditional communities. Ross McKibbin argues that the mother-daughter relationship was the axis of the working-class family.[38] In relation to London at the beginning of the twentieth century Ellen Ross has demonstrated that 'Mum' was the centre of the 'survival networks' by which extended families looked out for each other. It was 'Mum' who negotiated mutual assistance with other matriarchs in those larger networks which tied together neighbouring extended families.[39] Elizabeth Roberts depicted a similar matriarchal community in her oral history of Lancashire during the period 1890–1970.[40] In her analysis of working-class health culture, which was based on the same oral history interviews as Elizabeth Roberts' work, Lucinda Beier found that neighbours provided a long list of services to one another in terms of ill health including cooking, laundry, cleaning, childcare, errands, loans of supplies, provision of remedies, and laying out of the dead.[41] Whilst social changes, affluence and new housing did encourage the breakdown of these traditional matriarchal communities, in inner-city Liverpool, as late as the 1950s, Madeline Kerr found the attitude, 'I couldn't get on without my mother. I could get on without my husband. I don't notice him', was not unusual.[42] Whilst the Oxfordshire interviewees expressed concern that the extended family was declining due to the increasing mobility of its members they also felt that grandmothers were now perhaps playing a greater part in the provision of childcare than when their children were young, due to the increasing numbers of working mothers. Mavis thought grandmothers today, including herself, spent more time looking after their grandchildren than previous generations.[43]

This centrality of women within family and kinship networks was seen in relation to health. Experienced mothers, especially, developed expertise and authority regarding diagnosis and treatment of many ailments and offered advice to neighbours.[44] It was female health authorities that dominated the provision of care in the working-class Lancashire community that Lucinda Beier describes. She states that: 'There can be no doubt that working-class women were subordinate to working-class men. However, it is also true that working-class women were in charge at home and in neighbourhoods. Indeed, men essentially ceded control of these spaces to women by their absence.'[45] Therefore, it was women rather than men that were the central figures within the provision of lay medical care. Moreover, this female responsibility for health

---

38   McKibbin (1998), p. 170.
39   Ross (1983).
40   Roberts (1984); Roberts (1995).
41   Beier (2008), p. 52.
42   Kerr (1958), p. 40.
43   Mavis, EW10, p. 7.
44   Beier (2008), p. 54.
45   Beier (2008), p. 46.

care was not a new development. Margaret Pelling has shown that health care, like child care, seems perennially to have been a female responsibility.[46] Discussing the twentieth century Lucinda Beier argues that

> the expertise and authority of working-class women pervaded matters of health, governing dress, personal and home hygiene, diet, elimination, reproduction, disease prevention, diagnosis, therapeutics, first aid, nursing, and care of the dead. Female influence and agency regarding such issues were considered 'natural', associated with women's essential roles as nurturers of children and supporters of men.[47]

It was other women who featured most prominently in the accounts of the Oxfordshire women I have interviewed. Reminiscing about Benson life during her childhood in the 1940s, Gloria described the interdependency within the village which was based upon:

> Knowing families and knowing they're there if you need each other. I can see my mum now, we lived in the High Street and we were surrounded by elderly people, and no way would those people have been neglected. You didn't lock your doors or anything like that, you know if you were worried if they seemed ill or something, somebody would be in there to make sure they were okay.[48]

There was sadness in Gloria's account as she recalled what she felt was a vanishing world. This sense of loss was particularly upsetting as it highlighted the passing of a happy time in her life which may have caused her to exaggerate the villagers' closeness. However Gloria was reflecting on what has been viewed as a more general trend in respect to the breakdown of old communities and, associated with this, traditional health cultures. Commenting upon this change Lucinda Beier has posited that it resulted from the post-1945 welfare state which addressed the needs of the less prosperous and the increasing mobility which undermined the stability of working-class neighbourhoods and the long acquaintance and interdependence that had supported normative mutual aid. As a consequence Lucinda Beier believes that reliance on professional medicine and public health became both convenient and appropriate and by 1970, reached its zenith.[49]

However, by looking in more depth at the accounts of Oxfordshire women it is clear that women continued to rely on friends and kin as a source of knowledge on maternity and infant care. Interviewees stressed the value of the advice of other mothers whose knowledge resulted from the experience of raising their own children. Mothers, other relatives, and neighbours were continually referred to as sources of information. Discussing the return home from hospital after labour, in her study of childbirth in the late 1970s, Ann Oakley stated that, 'Homecoming is a time for mothers and daughters: nearly three-quarters of mothers gave practical help to their daughters at this time.'[50] Mothers were frequently referred to by the women I interviewed as having come to

46 Pelling (1997), p. 271.
47 Beier (2008), p. 35.
48 Gloria, BE14, pp. 21–22.
49 Beier (2008), pp. 27–28.
50 Oakley (1979), p. 147.

help them when their babies were born. This was perhaps particularly true for those women who lived in close proximity to their mothers. When talking about her sources of information on babycare, Siobhan, who was born in Abingdon and raised her children in nearby Benson, explained how, 'when I was young you just went and asked your mother.'[51] Gloria was born and brought up in Benson and had her own children in Benson in the mid 1960s. She strongly believed in the need for babies to have regular time outside in order to ensure they remained healthy: 'Don't matter if it was winter, or whatever, during the day for her sleep she'd be outside, both my babies. Wouldn't be in here, wouldn't be in her cot, she'd be in her pram, outside, under the plum tree, wrapped up snugly and warm if it was winter.' When asked why she thought it was important, she answered: 'It was something my mum used to do I suppose.'[52]

Tania lived in Hastings when her first baby was born in the 1950s and her mother lived around the corner. She thought that having her mother there 'did make a difference. She did give you confidence, which I think if she hadn't of been there, basically I might have gone to pieces.'[53] Moreover, for women, such as Tania, who had home-births, mothers were present during labour as well. Tania said her mother 'was with me on the three that I had at home, she was in and out the room'.[54] Tania had moved to Ewelme in between the births of her third and fourth babies and her mother had remained in Hastings. However, the move did not change the close relationship she enjoyed with her mother, and her mother came to stay with the family in Ewelme when Tania's fourth child was born. Indeed many interviewees who did not have their mothers living nearby still recalled them as being an important source of advice and knowledge. Telephones became an increasingly common means of keeping in touch. Claire was from London but lived in North Oxford when her children were born between 1962 and 1970. When asked why she followed a routine with her first baby she explained it was on the advice of her mother.[55] Maxine lived in Shipton-under-Wychwood and had three children in the late 1950s and early 1960s. She had grown up in Lancashire and therefore lived far away from her family, but still reported being influenced by her mother. When asked if she followed the advice of any childcare experts she replied: 'My mother followed the Truby King routine and gave me many tips.'[56] Sharon lived in Ewelme, a small village in south Oxfordshire when she had her children, while her mother lived in Liverpool. She recalled that she would turn to her mother for advice on how to care for her children. She ex-

51 Siobhan, BE1, pp. 26–27.
52 Gloria, BE14, p. 18.
53 Tania, EW8, p. 16.
54 Tania, EW8, p. 9.
55 Claire, NO1, p. 6.
56 Maxine, WY6, pp. 7–8.

plained how, 'Until the last couple of years before she died she was the person I could talk to about the children you know.'[57]

In addition, neighbours often filled the role of advice giver for women who did not live near their families. Grace lived in a small, private estate in Summertown, north Oxford when she had her first baby in the mid 1960s. She recalled her neighbour as being a hugely significant figure in her life, she would go to her neighbour with any questions about caring for her baby, and recalled her as being her 'salvation'.[58] Emily had three children in the 1960s. She lived in North Oxford, and was therefore at some distance from her family in Ireland. It was Emily's next-door neighbour who stepped into the role of confidant and guide. She explained that her neighbour 'had three children a little bit older, she was therefore an experienced mum [and] she really tutored me'.[59] Carol had the first of her five children as a teenage mother in the late 1970s and at the time was estranged from her own mother. She said two of her neighbours in Sandford where she was then living acted as 'parent role models' for her. She felt she learnt the practical aspects of childcare from one neighbour and about child development from the other.[60]

However while both friends and kin remained an essential source of advice for women it is noteworthy that husbands continued to play a more limited role. Pregnancy and childbirth were largely considered to be a female preserve well into the 1970s.[61] The husbands of women who had their children in the 1940s and 1950s were often forbidden from being present at the birth. Even during home-births many husbands chose to remain out of the room or were kept out by the midwives. Enid had her first baby at home in Benson in 1943. Her midwife sent her husband on a fictitious errand to Wallingford because she did not want him in the house.[62] Many of the women whose babies were born in the 1940s, 1950s and 1960s indicated ambivalence in their attitudes towards husbands being present. Interviewees whose husbands were not present often said they were glad he was not there. By the end of the 1960s this attitude had softened and men were increasingly encouraged to be present both during antenatal classes and hospital birth. Fiona felt her husband developed a closer relationship with their second son born in 1968 than with their first born in 1966 because he was present at the birth. She explained that he was 'more involved' because 'he'd been there and it wasn't this sort of women's mystery.'[63] By the early 1980s the father's presence at birth was part of established medical practice with fathers expected to support their labouring partners.[64] However, fathers were still expected to play a secondary

57   Sharon, EW9, p. 14.
58   Grace, NO7, p. 2.
59   Emily, NO8, p. 8.
60   Carol, TH14, p. 7.
61   Oakley (1979), p. 6.
62   Enid, BE12, p. 11.
63   Fiona, BE10, pp. 24–25.
64   Backett (1982), p. 73; Barbour (1990), p. 209.

and supportive role to mothers and this was reflected in the experience of the Oxfordshire women. Interviewees occasionally recalled consulting with their husbands, but the assumption childcare was ultimately the women's duty and the belief that mothers 'knew best' meant – at least during their children's infancy – that they were primarily responsible for deciding how to parent.

The advice of medical professionals

It is true, though, that despite women's continued reliance on family and friends, the role of medical professionals in providing advice about maternity and childcare was increasing. Whilst stressing that her mother was her first source of advice, Tania also told me that 'if there was anything wrong you went to the doctors.'[65] For Polly, whose children were born in Benson in the 1960s, her GP Dr Andrew Millar was her principal source of information. Indeed when asked whether she went to her mother for advice, she replied: 'Not really no. She was there obviously, but no, I put my faith I think in Andrew. As far as I was concerned he was a doctor and if he was happy with what was going on then so was I. Yes. As far as I was concerned it was Andrew who was the one I turned to.'[66] Fiona, also a Benson resident, described how when she brought her son home from hospital she went to her doctor with all her queries:

> To start with I went to the doctor. The doctor got a bit fed up with me. Cause poor little boy, October and I thought, well you have to keep babies warm. So the poor little devil got a heat rash. [Laughs.] Cause he had his woolly vest and his baby-grow and his woolly cardigan, so 'Perhaps, perhaps you should take some of these clothes off'. Which I thought, these strange spots what on earth are they? So anyway, I learnt my lesson after that.[67]

Many women wanted their doctors to provide more than a purely medical service and to fill the role of a confidant and source of advice. In the decades following the foundation of the NHS women were increasingly reliant on their GPs with greater expectations of the level of support they would receive. Most of the women did have good relations with their GP and these expectations were fulfilled, but if they were not women could feel let down.

For women who had home-births midwives also featured prominently in their accounts. The same midwife provided antenatal and postnatal care and also attended the delivery. Consequently a woman could build up a relationship with her midwife. For example Lisa who was living in Cowley when her baby was born, described how, 'I had the baby at home, the midwife came and delivered it [...] And then the midwife came in every day for the first week and then every other day for the next couple of weeks.'[68] Chloe Fisher

---

65   Tania, EW8, p. 17.
66   Polly, BE7, p. 13.
67   Fiona, BE10, p. 26.
68   Lisa, CO12, p. 10.

who worked in the city centre was a very well known figure and held in great affection.[69] For those women who had home-births, midwives could therefore fulfil the role of confidant and guide. However the relocation of birth from home to hospital that was occurring during the post-war years meant a decline in the importance of the independent midwife as the woman's attendant and therefore a change in the relationship between women and their midwives. The 1970 Peel report was a pivotal moment. Quickly after its release the rate of domiciliary delivery became negligible. Although at the great majority of deliveries the midwife remained the senior person present, the proportion of midwives with experience of home delivery continuously decreased. Midwives and their patients lost the continuing contact of home midwifery.[70] Those midwives who remained in the community became principally responsible for the postnatal care of women discharged early from hospital. While it would be wrong to dismiss the continued importance of the advice of midwives to mothers, interviewees who experienced hospital birth and then early discharge into the hands of their midwife, did not report the same close relationship with her as those who had undergone a home-birth. As Julia Allison has noted, from the 1970s the role of the geographically based midwife who offered a first point of contact with the maternity service faded into history.[71]

While the role of midwives as advice givers may have changed as the post-war years progressed, health visitors were continually referred to as an important source of advice. Indeed health visitors were expected to be the most significant figures in the lives of postnatal women. In 1960, the MOH for Oxfordshire M.J. Pleydell wrote: 'The health visitor with her knowledge and understanding [...] is a front-line worker in the promotion of mental and physical health.'[72] Some women did report their health visitors as being useful figures and the first person they would turn to if they had any questions or problems. Deborah, a Cowley resident, thought 'they were very nice people.'[73] Molly who lived in North Oxford reflected, 'It was nice having somebody come into the house, you know, and just talking to you while you'd got the baby on your lap, it was quite a nice atmosphere, and they seemed to be helpful.'[74] Karen felt that her health visitor was 'absolutely fantastic' and said, 'I've always been very grateful to her, because I knew absolutely nothing about babies at all and she managed to tell me all things I needed to know without making me feel like a complete fool for not knowing them.'[75] However other women resented the health visitor coming, thinking that she was interfering and passing judgment on their ability to care for their children. Grace was very uncomfortable

---

69   Chloe Fisher was referred to by Pippa, CO13, p. 10; Michelle, OX8, p. 7; Megan, OX11, p. 5; Lindsay, OX12, p. 11; Yvonne, NO3, p. 14; Tasha, SO14, p. 8; Kaye, WY14, p. 2.
70   Donnison (1977), p. 195; Campbell/Macfarlane (1994), p. 24.
71   Allison (1996), p. 111.
72   MOH Oxfordshire (1960), p. 13.
73   Deborah, CO6, p. 11.
74   Molly, NO4, p. 8.
75   Karen, SO4, p. 6.

when the health visitor came and presumed she was passing judgment upon her: 'I was pretty chaotic. We were living up the road in a little house which had one big room downstairs and these tiny babies and the health visitor used to come and visit invariably when the baby was sort of crawling round the floor in a filthy nappy.'[76] These ideas that health visitors were interfering, and that it was necessary to take their advice with a healthy scepticism, had been common in the inter-war years, and it is interesting that similar attitudes existed in the post-war period too.[77]

Indeed some women preferred to visit their local chemist rather than baby clinics staffed by health visitors. Chemists had traditionally provided the products that the baby clinics came to offer, such as baby foods, dummies and ointments and creams for nappy rash. Many chemists also provided a baby weighing service.[78] Before the advent of the NHS the local chemist was the obvious place to seek health care advice. When asked what health care was like when she was a child Olive, who was born in 1916, explained that, 'we used to go round to a people's dispensary in Marston Street […] I should think you know the care was reasonably good.'[79] Moreover this function of the chemist has remained even after the advent of the NHS and decline of financial barriers to consultation. Some people continued to view the chemist as the first step in primary care.[80] For example Deirdre who had her children in 1955 and 1958 chose to take her babies to be weighed in the chemist in Banbury where she used to work. Stuart Anderson and Virginia Berridge have argued that chemists and dispensaries operated in the middle-ground between traditional health sources and official medicine throughout the twentieth century. They demonstrate that,

> local chemists have had strong links with the traditions of lay care and with popular medicine: they have been a readily accessible and unpaid source of health information, advice and support. They have been available in most communities throughout Great Britain, over extended hours and without appointment, providing advice on a wide range of health matters without charge.

What is also interesting about these chemists is that unlike community health authorities, most chemists were men.[81] However, women could still be an important presence within the shops. Fanny, who had two children in Oxford in the 1960s, recalled it was the chemist's wife who was her main source of information on childcare. She explained,

> We had a very good chemist along the road […] and it was a chemist and his wife and his wife had been a nurse and I got as much advice from her about kids than anyone, and she, she used to tell me all sorts, 'You must talk to them, even if you don't they know what

---

76   Grace, NO7, pp. 1–2.
77   Graham Smith found this scepticism amongst women in his study of mothers in Dundee between 1911 and 1931. Smith (1995), p. 66.
78   Anderson/Berridge (2000), p. 62.
79   Olive, OX6, p. 13.
80   Beier (2008), p. 92.
81   Anderson/Berridge (2000), p. 48.

you're talking about, you must talk to them', and all sorts of things. And they had, I used to get the food there and the baby food until they were older.[82]

As well as their midwives, health visitors, GPs and chemists women also sought advice from childcare literature. For example, several of the interviewees explained that they put their faith in Dr Benjamin Spock, author of the famous "Baby and Childcare", rather than seeking advice from their mothers. Camilla stated that she 'was the Spock generation' and 'didn't believe in old wives' tales'. She felt her generation were consequently better parents: 'my generation was quite lucky in being given a bit more advice in the upbringing of their children rather than listening to mother.'[83] Similarly Lindsay preferred to follow the advice of Benjamin Spock than her mother, even though her mother was a doctor, because she thought her mother was too old-fashioned. Lindsay was therefore not turning away from old wives' talks in favour of medical expertise, rather her rejection of her mother's advice was indicative of a clash of generations. She told me: 'Mother was a strong advocate of potty training from I think three months. I was going by Spock and took the view there was no point in trying to potty train before the child knew what the hell was going on.'[84]

Lucinda Beier has also referred to this generational shift in attitudes with reference to the oral history interviews she and Elizabeth Roberts conducted in Lancashire for the period 1890–1970. Lucinda Beier states, 'As the "modern" generation, born after 1920, came of age, working-class health culture was increasingly regarded as quaint and backward – associated with gendered ignorance and superstition, encapsulated in "old wives' tales" and displayed in a variety of unhealthy behaviors.'[85] I would like to suggest that this difference between the generations may also have been a result of the younger generation wanting to assert their independence and own authority as mothers. Indeed this generation gap between mothers and daughters was also seen in the relationship between women and medical professionals as well. Ian Tait and Susanna Graham-Jones argue that:

> The 'generation gap' in post-war Britain illustrated a major shift in family life and in society at large [...] In the flamboyant atmosphere of the 1960s, for the generation which, in Harold Macmillan's phrase, had 'never had it so good', the old deference for authority figures such as parents, grandparents, doctors, and teachers seemed outdated and unnecessary. Doctor-patient relationships – like other relationships – became much less formal in the space of one generation.[86]

82 Fanny, OX4, p. 15.
83 Camilla, SO6, p. 11.
84 Lindsay, OX12, pp. 14–15.
85 Beier (2004), p. 409.
86 Tait/Graham-Jones (1998), p. 236.

Professional expertise versus personal experience

I would also like to argue that in turning to medical professionals women were not simply rejecting the knowledge of their mothers and other lay women. I think that as important was their desire to seek a replacement for mothers who were not around, or whom they did not get on with. Sometimes neighbours would do. When they were not available, or considered unsuitable, doctors could also be consulted. Lucinda Beier has argued that 'the status of the health care professionals was quite different from that of neighbors' because 'their authority stemmed from their credentials rather than from their personal reputations in the neighborhood'.[87] However, from the interviews with Oxfordshire women I found that in respect to advice surrounding maternity and childcare, it was not their professional credentials that were most valued, but rather their own experience of parenthood.

This value attributed to parenthood was evident in the case of Dr Anne Millar, a GP in Benson. Although when Anne Millar originally came to Benson it was solely in the role of doctor's wife she gradually became more involved in the practice. Having a female doctor who was a mother and someone the women felt was approachable was a constantly mentioned and obviously important fact for the women. It was Anne Millar who ran the baby clinic in the village. She was considered a good source of advice, and was someone the women felt they could trust. Siobhan explained that,

> if I'd ever had any doubts about it, there was Dr Anne here in the village and she was absolutely fantastic. She gave you a lot of confidence in how you were doing. She ran a clinic and you could take your child along and have it checked to make sure everything was ok. And she was incredibly reassuring and encouraging and you just felt that if things weren't right she'd tell you, and it gave you a lot of confidence so yeah, we were lucky.[88]

Many of the Benson interviewees felt they established a good rapport with her and she was well liked. What I think is interesting is that the interviewees held Anne Millar's knowledge as a mother in as high regard as they did her professional knowledge as a doctor. Ellen specifically mentioned the fact she was a mother as being why she valued her advice. She thought she was a 'very practical, sensible woman. She'd got older children, but you got the feeling she knew what she was talking about. She's been through the same sort of thing.'[89] In turning to Anne Millar the Benson women were not indicating that they viewed expertise in maternity and childcare as being the preserve of health professionals. They were not supporting the discourse of medical authority. They consulted her because they thought she could offer advice in her capacity as an experienced mother. Her professional knowledge may have augmented this, but it could not replace it.

87   Beier (2008), p. 80.
88   Siobhan, BE1, p. 17.
89   Ellen, EW3, p. 5.

It was also Dr Anne Millar's personal experience of parenthood rather than simply her gender that was valued. Male doctors who were parents were also favoured. Shula had three children in a small north Oxfordshire village in the late 1960s and early 1970s. She explained that she had excellent care from her male GP, who 'had three young children, very similar to us, you know about a year older'.[90] It was not only doctors, but also other health professionals with children of their own who were preferred. Pippa had three children in the 1980s. She explained that once she had children she chose to see a female doctor with children of her own because, she 'felt empathy there because she clearly loved babies', adding that 'interestingly [...] I felt the health visitors who had their own children were better'.[91] Interviewees also indicated their scepticism about the advice of medical professionals who did not have children. For example, Nina, who had two children in Thame in the mid 1970s, said, 'With my first one the health visitor was a mother herself and she was brilliant and she was older, so she was a real help. But the second one it was a young, just trained, she hadn't got a clue, she used to ask me what I thought and that was no help at all. So I think if they've actually been through it themselves they can be of more use.'[92] Alma, who had twins in Thame in the mid 1980s stated that: 'I think they should advertise for health visitors who have to have children of their own, that would be very sensible.'[93] Bev had two children in 1987 and 1990 and was even more explicit in her dissatisfaction of her health visitor saying, 'I found her dead useless because she had never had children herself.'[94] Midwives who had not had their own children also faced criticism. Sandra was unhappy with the midwives who attended her in hospital, calling them, 'really old-fashioned spinsters who had no idea what it was like'.[95] Andrea had her first baby in 1978. She said her midwife

> was not married and she hasn't had children and a lot of it she was reading out the textbook but she didn't have the experience. And even afterwards she didn't have the experience of what it was like to be up all night with a crying baby. So I mean I have to [...] coz my youngest daughter is actually a paediatric nurse and if I could have had her around, it's well we've done the same training but it's sometimes experience, you can't teach experience.[96]

Conclusion

By examining oral history accounts of women's experiences of motherhood in the post-war decades this paper has tried to show how despite the social

---

90 Shula, BA12, p. 7.
91 Pippa, CO13, pp. 10–11.
92 Nina, TH3, pp. 11–12.
93 Alma, TH7, pp. 11–12.
94 Bev, CR10, p. 12.
95 Sandra, EW13, p. 6.
96 Andrea, SA9, p. 4.

changes seen since 1945 and the introduction of the NHS in 1948, mothers have continued to value the advice of experienced parents in respect to maternity and childcare. Firstly, their continued reliance on the advice of both friends and kin was demonstrated. Then, I showed that issues of generational conflict could be as important as a positive desire for biomedical knowledge in explaining women's rejection of their own mothers' advice. Finally, I have argued that even when mothers did turn to orthodox medicine, they could still value the practical experience of the caregiver over their professional expertise. Lucinda Beier has argued that, 'As the elderly neighbourhood authorities on ill health, childbearing, and death retired or died in the post-War period, no one took their place.'[97] I would like to suggest that there was someone taking the place – medical professionals. GPs, health visitors and others were in many ways the direct heirs of the neighbourhood authorities, providing the same functions. Discussing the role of the GP in the 1980s Cecil Helman has argued that:

> Contrary to its original intention, the NHS in Britain may have reinforced the 'folk healer' aspect of its GPs; a much wider range of life experience and misfortune is now being dealt with by GPs – not only a wider range of illness and disease than formerly but also psychological crises, life crises (such as bereavement, divorce, etc.), and all the normal biological landmarks, such as birth, childhood, puberty, menopause and death.[98]

Similarly, I do not think that by turning to medical professionals women were renouncing the traditional advice based on experience they had previously received from kin. Rather than seeking information from the GPs, health visitors and others simply because of their familiarity with biomedicine, women valued those professionals with practical experience of parenthood. The women I interviewed continued to respect the know-how of lay sources such as friends and kin. While they may have supplemented this with medical advice when they felt it was needed, there was no wholesale rejection of traditional knowledge.

Bibliography

The Agricultural Economics Research Institute Oxford: Country Planning: A Study of Rural Problems. London 1944.

Allison, Julia: Delivered at Home. London 1996.

Anderson, Stuart; Berridge, Virginia: The Role of the Community Pharmacist in Health and Welfare 1911–1986. In: Bornat, Joanna; Perks, Robert; Thompson, Paul; Walmsley, Jan (eds.): Oral History, Health and Welfare. London 2000, pp. 48–74.

Backett, Kathryn C.: Mothers and Fathers: A Study of the Development and Negotiation of Parental Behaviour. London 1982.

Barbour, Rosaline S.: Fathers: The Emergence of a New Consumer Group. In: Garcia, Jo; Kilpatrick, Robert; Richards, Martin (eds.): The Politics of Maternity Care. Oxford 1990, pp. 202–216.

97 Beier (2001), p. 236.
98 Helman (1986), p. 231.

Beier, Lucinda McCray: 'I Used to Take Her to the Doctor and Get the *Proper* Thing': Twenti-
    eth-Century Health Care Choices in Lancashire Working-Class Communities. In: Shirley,
    Michael H.; Larson, Todd E.A. (eds.): Splendidly Victorian: Essays in Nineteenth- and
    Twentieth-Century British History in Honour of Walter L. Arnstein. Aldershot 2001,
    pp. 221–241.
Beier, Lucinda McCray: Expertise and Control: Childbearing in Three Twentieth-Century
    Working-Class Lancashire Communities. In: Bulletin of the History of Medicine 78 (2004),
    no. 2, pp. 379–409.
Beier, Lucinda McCray: For Their Own Good: The Transformation of English Working-Class
    Health Culture, 1880–1970. Columbus 2008.
Bourke, Joanna: Working-Class Cultures in Britain 1890–1960: Gender, Class and Ethnicity.
    London 1994.
Campbell, Rona; Macfarlane, Alison: Where to Be Born? The Debate and the Evidence. Ox-
    ford 1994.
Campbell, Stephen M.; Roland, Martin O.: Why Do People Consult the Doctor? In: Family
    Practice 13 (1996), pp. 75–83.
Carr-Hill, Roy A.; Rice, Nigel; Roland, Martin: Socioeconomic Determinants of Rates of
    Consultation in General Practice Based on Fourth National Morbidity Survey of General
    Practices. In: British Medical Journal 312 (1996), pp. 1008–1012.
Cartwright, Ann: Patients and Their Doctors. London 1967.
Cartwright, Ann; Anderson, Robert: General Practice Revisited: A Second Study of Patients
    and Their Doctors. London 1981.
City of Oxford: Annual Reports of the Medical Officer of Health. Bodleian Library.
Cornwell, Jocelyn: Hard-Earned Lives: Accounts of Health and Illness from East London.
    London 1984.
Davis, Angela: Motherhood in Oxfordshire, c. 1945–1970: A Study of Attitudes, Experiences
    and Ideals. DPhil Thesis Oxford 2007.
Department of Health and Social Security: Report of the Sub-Committee on Domiciliary and
    Maternity Bed Needs. London 1970.
Digby, Anne: The Evolution of British General Practice, 1850–1948. Oxford 1999.
Donnison, Jean: Midwives and Medical Men: A History of Inter-Professional Rivalries and
    Women's Rights. New York 1977.
Field, Katherine: Children of the Nation?: A Study of the Health and Well-being of Oxford-
    shire Children, 1891–1939. DPhil Thesis Oxford 2001.
Fisher, Kate: An Oral History of Birth Control Practice c. 1925–50: A Study of Oxford and
    South Wales. DPhil Thesis Oxford 1997.
Hardy, Ann: Health and Medicine in Britain since 1860. Houndmills, Basingstoke 2001.
Helman, Cecil G.: 'Feed a Cold, Starve a Fever': Folk Models of Infection in an English Sub-
    urban Community, and their Relation to Medical Treatment. In: Currer, Caroline; Stacey,
    Margaret (eds.): Concepts of Health, Illness and Disease: A Comparative Perspective. Ox-
    ford 1986, pp. 213–231.
Jones, Helen: Health and Society in Twentieth-Century Britain. London 1994.
Kapur, Navneet; Hunt, Isabelle; Lunt, Mark; McBeth, John; Creed, Francis; Macfarlane,
    Gary: Primary Care Consultation Predictors in Men and Women: A Cohort Study. In:
    British Journal of General Practice 55 (2005), pp. 108–113.
Kerr, Madeline: The People of Ship Street. London 1958.
McKibbin, Ross: Classes and Cultures: England 1918–1951. Oxford 1998.
Ministry of Health: Report of the Maternity Services Committee. London 1959.
Möller-Leimkuhler, Anne Maria: Barriers to Help-Seeking by Men: A Review of Sociocul-
    tural and Clinical Literature with Particular Reference to Depression. In: Journal of Affec-
    tive Disorders 71 (2002), pp. 1–9.
Oakley, Ann: Becoming a Mother. Oxford 1979.

Oxfordshire County Council: Annual Reports of the County Medical Officer of Health and Principal School Medical Officer. Centre for Oxfordshire Studies.

Parfit, Jessie: The Health of a City: Oxford, 1770–1974. Oxford 1987.

Pelling, Margaret: Unofficial and Unorthodox Medicine. In: Loudon, Irvine (ed.): The Oxford Illustrated History of Western Medicine. Oxford 1997, pp. 264–276.

Peretz, Elizabeth: The Costs of Modern Motherhood to Low Income Families in Interwar Britain. In: Fildes, Valerie; Marks, Lara; Marland, Hilary (eds.): Women and Children First: International Maternal and Child Welfare 1870–1945. London 1992, pp. 257–280.

Rice, Margery Spring: Working-Class Wives: Their Health and Conditions. Harmondsworth 1939.

Roberts, Elizabeth: A Woman's Place: An Oral History of Working-Class Women, 1890–1940. Oxford 1984.

Roberts, Elizabeth: Women and Families: An Oral History, 1940–1970. Oxford 1995.

Ross, Ellen: Survival Networks: Women's Neighbourhood Sharing in London before the First World War. In: History Workshop Journal 15 (1983), pp. 4–27.

Scaife, Brett; Gill, Paramjit S.; Heywood, Phillip L.; Neal, Richard D.: Socio-Economic Characteristics of Adult Frequent Attenders in General Practice: Secondary Analysis of Data. In: Family Practice 17 (2000), pp. 298–304.

Smith, Graham: Protest is Better for Infants: Motherhood, Health and Welfare in a Woman's Town, c. 1911–1931. In: Oral History 23 (1995), pp. 63–70.

Steedman, Carolyn: Landscape of a Good Woman: The Story of Two Lives. London 1986.

Summerfield, Penny: Reconstructing Women's Wartime Lives. Manchester 1998.

Tait, Ian; Graham-Jones, Susanna: General Practice, its Patients and the Public. In: Loudon, Irvine; Horder, John; Webster, Charles (eds.): General Practice under the National Health Service. London 1998, pp. 224–246.

Verbrugge, Lois M.: The Twain Meet: Empirical Explanations of Sex Differences in Health and Mortality. In: Journal of Health and Social Behavior 30 (1989), pp. 282–304.

'Mother knows best'. The transmission of knowledge of the female body and venereal diseases in nineteenth-century Dutch rape cases*

Willemijn Ruberg

Introduction

This chapter analyses how knowledge of the female body was constructed, transmitted and negotiated in nineteenth-century Dutch rape cases. It is part of an ongoing research project on Dutch forensic medicine in the eighteenth and nineteenth centuries. Before the late nineteenth century, forensic medicine was not an institutionalized discipline. From about 1840 texts were published advocating a professionalization of forensic medicine in the Netherlands.[1] It was only in the nineteenth century that Dutch textbooks on forensic medicine were published; before that period, and still during most of the nineteenth century, foreign books were consulted, mostly German texts. However, the lack of professionalization of Dutch forensic medicine did not mean that doctors were not consulted in lawsuits. Sometimes judges requested medical examinations of victims, more often the relatives of the victims (many of the rape victims were children) took the initiative to look for a physician who could corroborate the victim's experience. What is more, knowledge of the body was not limited to physicians. Before the nineteenth century, midwives were also responsible for examining women's bodies when it came to pregnancy or rape. In this chapter I will argue that laywomen's knowledge, especially that of the mothers of rape victims, played an important part in the construction of forensic knowledge of the body.

Before I will elaborate on the advantages and limits of my archival sources, I will sketch which insights from recent work on the history and sociology of knowledge have helped to shape my approach to these sources. Firstly, feminist epistemology has pointed out that women's knowledge has often been disqualified as not being 'real' knowledge. If knowledge is defined as an individual's command of learned facts, women's knowledge often does not count since it is frequently based on (individual or collective) experience, not written down, or collectively established.[2] We might expand this insight to include the knowledge of the lower classes, inferiors or outsiders in general. In addition, feminist epistemology showed that knowledge can never be objective or universal, but is always 'situated'. Some feminist standpoint theorists concluded

* I would like to thank professor Hilary Marland for her helpful comments on a previous version of this essay.
1 Broecke/Broecke (1845).
2 Alcoff/Potter (1993); Potter (1993); Hekman (1997).

that women's points of view were more 'real' because women were oppressed. Poststructuralist feminist theorists, however, criticized this view as being essentialist and emphasized that knowledge was always socially constructed.

Secondly, in regard to the history of knowledge, historians of the early modern period recently emphasized that the production of knowledge is 'a social process, that includes many different communities of practitioners'.[3] Knowledge making has a collective nature and involves the agency of historical actors. The question then is: which historical actors possessed knowledge of the body and who had the authority to disseminate this knowledge? Historians have often shown how, especially in the nineteenth century, the male medical profession acquired its position at the cost of traditional midwives.[4] In this history, there is neither a role for a negotiation of knowledge, nor attention to the role of the patient or the family, whereas I would like to focus on exactly these elements. Historians of doctor-patient relationships have indicated how in the eighteenth and early nineteenth centuries, patients and doctors often used the same discourse, a mixture between medical and lay terms. Laymen also actively participated in medicine, for instance in gentlemen's magazines, as Roy Porter has shown.[5] This points to the fact that there might not have been a very big gap between the medical knowledge of doctors and lay people.[6] Moreover, Nancy Theriot has considered how doctors, patients and families negotiated illness in the nineteenth century. While the physician needed the patient to formulate her life story and therefore left some aspects to her discretion, he, at the same time, steered questions to her based on his medical expertise. Theriot argues that female patients helped construct scientific medical knowledge.[7] Similarly, medical anthropologists have emphasized that the boundaries between lay people and doctors are continually shifting, laypersons sometimes acquiring medical knowledge, while doctors are often laymen compared to medical specialists.[8]

In my research into nineteenth-century Dutch rape cases, I study how knowledge of the body was negotiated between physicians, midwives, lawyers, judges, witnesses, victims and their families, who together formed a (micro) 'health care system'. In this chapter, I will specifically address the role of the mother of the rape victim. A majority of rape victims were young girls and their mothers played a big part in the accusation. I will focus on the transmission of the mother's knowledge of her daughter's body: was this knowledge taken seriously by medical doctors? If so, was this knowledge then collectively created? Bypassing the question of which knowledge is 'more true', I assume

---

3   Smith/Schmidt (2007), p. 7. See also Porter/Hall (1995).
4   Dalmiya/Alcoff (1993); Borg (1992), pp. 144–145.
5   Porter: Lay medical knowledge (1985).
6   See for example Duden (1991); Stolberg (2003); Porter: Patient's view (1985).
7   Theriot (2001), p. 361.
8   Willems (1992), p. 105.

not only that all knowledge is socially constructed, but also shared and negotiated.[9]

Archives and sources

Doctors' reports on physical examinations are sometimes part of court files, depending on what elements of these archives have been kept. Also in testimonies of victims, perpetrators and witnesses, remarks on bodies and medicine can be found. However, as many historians have pointed out, legal sources cannot be taken at face value. All testimonies were responses to questions from police officers, judges or mayors, so they were heavily steered and structured by the goals of these officials. In addition, we have to take into account that these stories were shaped according to cultural conventions, legal restraints, audiences and the personal interests of victims, perpetrators and witnesses, as Garthine Walker has demonstrated for early modern English cases of rape.[10] A specific problem with the Dutch sources is the absence of an explicit account of the impact of medical testimony. They hardly ever specified to what extent the physician's opinion on the occurrence of rape determined the outcome of the trial. The historian can only infer this by comparing the evidence given and the final verdict. However, I am not so much interested in the relative weight of the voice of the forensic doctor, as in the preceding process of negotiation of medical knowledge.

The court archives I studied are those of the consecutive provincial courts of law, that pronounced judgment on serious crimes such as murder and violent rape. Two sections in the law addressed 'facts against the honour of a girl younger than fifteen, executed with violence'. Of the 140 rape cases I studied in the archives of the provincial courts of North Holland, dating from 1813–1884, 68 cases (49%) involved children under 15, mostly girls (although there were four cases of adult men raping young boys). I also found four cases of incest, two of which concerned children under 15 years of age. Since many of the other cases featured children between 15 and 18 years of age, the number of cases of child rape would be much higher if we applied our contemporary definition of childhood. These legal documents provide information about the lower classes' attitudes towards sexuality, violence and the body, since the victims and perpetrators nearly always belonged to this social stratum.

---

9   Also see Jordanova (1995); Burke (2000).
10   Walker (1998), pp. 3–5.

Signs on the body

Since nearly half of all rape cases concerned children, the mother was involved, too. The role of the mother when it comes to the interpretation of
signs on children's bodies has not been studied very often. In the majority of
rape cases the parents took their children to see a doctor, after the child had
told them what had happened and the mother had inspected the body first. In
two cases it was the medical doctor who, after having examined the child, advised the parents to bring charges against the perpetrator. Often, the Chief
Constable or magistrate then ordered another physician to examine the child.
It also happened that parents were sent to a physician with their child directly
after they had lodged their complaint. Only in one case the examination was
carried out by an almost illiterate midwife. Doctors who wrote textbooks of
forensic medicine were rather condescending about the 'expertise' of midwives.[11] They claimed midwives were not to be trusted.

The discovery of rape, however, had often started with the mother. In
nearly all of these cases, girls confessed to their mothers that they had been
raped or sexually assaulted. Often, this confession was not easy for the girl.
The mother had to extract it because the girl felt ashamed or because she was
afraid her mother would punish her for seeing boys, which was often forbidden. So the mother was someone a child could confide in, but also a parent
who had the potential to punish. In many cases, the mother then went on to
examine her daughter's body. She looked at the genitals, but the child's clothes
were also scrutinized for signs of violence (tears) or stains indicating bodily
fluids like blood, semen, or pus. Since women always did the laundry, they
could exercise social control by keeping track of bodily changes of relatives.
Women knew which women in the extended household menstruated or had
white discharge and they recognized spots of semen on clothes or bed linen
and venereal discharges.

When mothers examined their daughter's clothes while doing the laundry
or after their daughter had notified them of the sexual assault, they had to interpret the stains or fluids found. For instance, a mother had to distinguish
between normal white vaginal discharge and stains of semen. Mothers also
had to decide whether blood stains derived from a sexual assault or from the
child's normal scratching. After the rape of her fourteen-year-old daughter, a
mother was interrogated and asked if she had examined her daughter's body
and her undergarments and shirt.[12] She had not, but the question itself reveals
that the authorities expected a mother to perform these examinations. In other
cases as well, assumptions about the close relationship between mother and
daughter become apparent. An eighteen-year-old girl remained timid after
her sexual assault had been disclosed and 'was very surly even to her mother'.[13]

---

11 Koster (1877), p. 23; Meersch Bosch (1814), p. 253.
12 Noord-Hollands Archief (hereafter NHA), Provinciaal Gerechtshof Noord-Holland
    (hereafter PGNH), inv. no. 351, 4 February 1867.
13 NHA, Hof van Assisen (hereafter AHA), inv. no. 533, 9 April 1835.

In another case, the police noted down that a mother was prepared to declare under oath that her daughter was an honourable girl who had never been with a man.[14]

Mothers were supposed to know the character and behaviour of their children, as well as their bodies. The fact that mothers also scrutinized their children's clothes after an attack indicated that they were looking for proof of violence, but might also be explained by referring to prevailing conceptions of the body. Historians of the body have pointed out that the early modern period did not recognize a separation between the skin and garments as we now know it. Laura Gowing has termed clothing in seventeenth-century England as some kind of second skin: 'Early modern bodies were [...] covered in layers of inner and outer garments that were worn so long they were likely to become part of both the visible self, and inner subjectivity.'[15] Barbara Duden pointed out in her study of female patients of an eighteenth-century German doctor how these women experienced a completely different boundary between inner and outer body than we would do today: 'the skin does not appear as a material seal shutting the inside off from the outside. Instead it was a collection of real, minute orifices – the pores – and potential larger openings.'[16] Whereas in the early modern period, physicians hardly ever inspected the body, but relied on patients' descriptions of pain or bodily changes, from the nineteenth century doctors started to examine the body. However, in the nineteenth century many medical beliefs and habits coexisted with more 'modern' beliefs. One of these was the importance attached to clothes as a second skin. Although mothers and physicians in most cases examined the body itself, there are also a few cases in which the mother examined the clothes and undergarments, but not the body.[17]

Women's inspection of their daughters' clothes, in addition to their knowledge of the girls' bodily functioning based on doing the laundry, were particularly useful when it came to the recognition of venereal diseases. I have found a total of five cases where the victims became infected with a venereal disease after the assault. In the earliest case, dating from 1819, although the victim had genital warts, the accused was not ordered to undergo a physical examination and was acquitted.[18] In the four other cases, dating from 1822 until 1860, the accused was examined as well, and in three of these cases he was found to have the same venereal disease as the child and was convicted.[19] In one case, the accused was found not to have a venereal disease, but he was convicted on different grounds.[20] Although prostitutes were always seen as the sources of

14   NHA, PGNH, inv. no. 82, 17 October 1842.
15   Gowing (2003), p. 34.
16   Duden (1991), pp. 48, 121.
17   NHA, PGNH, inv. no. 104, 30 July 1844.
18   NHA, AHA, inv. no. 223, 26 July 1819.
19   NHA, AHA, inv. nos. 283, 496; NHA, PGNH, inv. no. 293.
20   NHA, PGNH, inv. no. 297, 4 October 1860.

infection with syphilis and gonorrhoea[21], disregarding the infection by male customers, from at least 1822 in the cases of child rape, the male perpetrator was regarded as the source of infection. These results are very different from Louise Jackson's study on child rape in Victorian England. Jackson found many doctors refused to see venereal disease as sexually transmitted and saw mothers or children as lying about it and trying to trick doctors.[22]

Mothers could play a part in establishing the connection between perpetrator and victim by way of a common venereal disease. For example, in 1822 a mother discovered that her eight-year-old daughter's genitalia secreted a badly smelling discharge, mixed with blood. She first thought the girl had started menstruating at a very young age, but later noticed the same discharge on the linen of her brother-in-law, who suffered from a venereal disease. The maid had noticed this as well. She found this suspicious, but the court records mention that this evidence did not support definitive conclusions.[23] The mother requested a physician to examine her daughter and he concluded she was suffering from gonorrhoea. The mother had picked this particular physician, although he was not the one they normally consulted, because she thought he was treating her brother-in-law for a venereal disease. She had consulted another doctor first, but since he had concluded the child was not suffering from a venereal disease, she had decided to go to another physician.

Although mothers often wanted doctors to corroborate the sexual abuse, which testifies to the physicians' respected authority, women also had considerable agency when it came to choosing a doctor, as the last case shows. In a similar case from 1859, a five-year-old girl was sexually assaulted by her uncle, a sailor who lived with the family. Four weeks before the assault her mother (the sailor's sister) had noticed when washing her brother's shirts traces of 'a secret disease'. So when a doctor concluded that her little daughter was suffering from gonorrhoea, the mother's knowledge made the connection to the perpetrator easier. In court, the physician testified the mother had told him she had found blood on the child's genitals, as well as semen stains on her shirt.[24] Not only did the doctor take this mother's knowledge seriously, he also reported the assault to the police on the basis of his examination and the information provided by the mother. In this case, the physician's knowledge appears to have been built on the mother's knowledge.

The question is whether, in general, women's knowledge was taken seriously. On the whole it was, since it was included in the case records and often not questioned. In a few cases, physicians were of the opinion that women were wrong. For instance, in 1851 a sixteen-year-old servant girl was raped. A female neighbour made her undress in front of her to see if she could find evidence of the assault. When questioned later, she claimed that the girl's shirt and underpants contained traces of semen. A physician who had examined

21   See Mooij (1993), p. 38.
22   Jackson (2000), pp. 76–77; see also Robertson (2005), pp. 50–52.
23   NHA, AHA, inv. no. 283, 22 April 1822.
24   NHA, PGNH, inv. no. 293, 20 October 1859.

the girl before, however, stated that he had not found any traces of semen (nor other bodily evidence).[25] The court records mention that therefore the earlier testimony of the woman did not have any value. The final verdict emphasized that the doctor, not the widow, was to be believed concerning the stains; it referred to his examination that had not detected any injuries; it mentioned that the girl testified in court to having had pain, whereas she had denied this when the physician had asked her; lastly it was pointed out that the tears in her panties need not necessarily have been caused by the defendant who was acquitted. In this particular case medical opinion overruled a common woman's view.

Medical techniques

Although it seems that in general medical doctors and judges listened and valued women's knowledge of the child's body, this was affected by the use that was made of medical technology requiring specific expertise. Empirical philosopher Annemarie Mol argued in her ethnographic study "The body multiple" (2002) that medical objects such as bodies and diseases only come into being with the practices used to study them and that each technique conveys a different picture resulting in multiple realities of the body:

> knowledge is not understood as a matter of reference, but as one of manipulation. The driving question is no longer 'how to find the truth?' but 'how are objects handled in practice?' With this shift, the philosophy of knowledge acquires an *ethnographic* interest in knowledge practices.[26]

Applying Mol's *praxiographic* approach, one technique that comes to the fore in Dutch nineteenth-century rape cases is the use of microscopes. Physicians employed microscopes to study (semen) stains on clothes. In textbooks of forensic medicine, the role of the microscope in analysing stains was increasingly mentioned in the second half of the nineteenth century.[27] In the source material I have studied, physicians used microscopes from 1860.[28] Under a microscope, doctors saw a completely different body than mothers or other lay persons did when they observed the body with the naked eye.

Another example of techniques producing different bodies is the examination of the hymen. Whereas mothers never looked for presence or absence of the hymen, midwives (until the nineteenth century) and doctors did touch the body internally, mostly inserting a finger in the vagina. This 'technique' also made the image, and thus the knowledge, diverge that doctors and mothers had of the body.

25   NHA, PGNH, inv. no. 44, 25 September 1851.
26   Mol (2002), p. 5.
27   Bergmann (1848), p. 362.
28   NHA, PGNH, inv. nos. 297, 25 October 1861; 309, 4 October 1861.

The hymen is one of the most discussed body parts in history and carries a significant symbolic burden. Especially religious authorities have established many rules and explanations surrounding virginity.[29] Textbooks on forensic medicine for centuries devoted chapters to the establishment of virginity. These textbooks, instructing physicians on what kinds of examinations to perform on victims and bodies, offered a list of signs relevant to detect rape. They paid much attention to signs of virginity, including full, red and tight labia, a narrow and wrinkled vagina, a short clitoris with a protruding foreskin, firm breasts and an intact hymen. Although nineteenth-century doctors no longer believed in ancient signs of virginity like dark nipples, murky urine, a hoarse voice or a thick neck, and although they acknowledged that none of the signs were conclusive, they still devoted long chapters to signs indicating virginity. For instance, they knew the hymen could have been ruptured before the first intercourse (by jumping or horse riding), and they were also aware of cases in which the hymen stayed intact after intercourse. Yet, they clung to these signs as indicators of virginity.

When comparing these theoretical statements to the practical examinations during rape trials, we see that tracing virginity does not seem to have been the most important task for physicians. Since nearly all the cases I studied concerned conviction on the basis of article 331, indecent assault performed *by force*, what was of equal or greater importance was finding proof of violence committed during the (attempted) rape. So, any signs on the body indicating violence were relevant. Still, inspection of the genitals including the hymen did occur. I have found seven cases in which doctors searched for the hymen (but in a number of cases extensive records no longer exist, so the incidence of medical examinations could be higher). In 1827, for example, a nine-year-old girl was examined only a few hours after she had been assaulted by a physician who authoritatively stated that the girl's genitals had been violated by someone's finger, causing a broken hymen and a considerable haemorrhage, still bleeding during the examination. The accused was convicted to half an hour in the pillory and six years confinement in a house of correction.[30]

However, not all cases were as clear-cut as this one as a second example will show. In 1861 a fourteen-year-old servant girl claimed to have been raped. The first doctor who examined her merely concluded he thought it was highly probable that intercourse had taken place. The magistrate thought this medical report did not suffice and ordered an examination by a second physician who wrote in his report:

> From what I found, although lacking more certain evidence, I have concluded a high probability of intercourse having taken place, although I cannot be certain since the hymen is often also broken by coincidence, without intercourse, or its opening is naturally wide.[31]

29   Adelman (2009).
30   NHA, AHA, inv. no. 397, 1 October 1827.
31   NHA, PGNH, inv. no. 305, 6 August 1861.

This medical doctor professed his uncertainty in regard to the bodily signs. In another case, the medical experts differed from one another. In 1814 a nine-year-old Jewish girl in Amsterdam was sexually assaulted by a 59-year-old man who put his finger in her vagina. Her grandfather, with whom she and her mother lived, immediately sent for a physician, who concluded that her genitals were heavily inflamed and the hymen was broken. The magistrate, however, ordered another physical examination and appointed three doctors, one a professor, to perform it. They claimed the girl's external genitals looked normal, but her internal genitals were red and swollen, whereas the hymen was present.[32] Interestingly, these three doctors disagreed with the first one who had thought the hymen was ruptured. The accused was acquitted but it is unclear why. Probably because it had not been proved conclusively that the defendant had used violence, a condition for conviction under article 331. However, one might speculate that the disagreement amongst the medical doctors did not help the case. What is more, the one doctor who thought the hymen was broken was Jewish, like the victim. Possibly, prejudice worked against the Jews, and in favour of the gentile doctors.

In any case, what stands out in many cases is the sheer uncertainty in regard to the bodily signs of rape. Generally, when a medical doctor stated there had not been any intercourse, or there had been intercourse but it was unclear if it had been rape, and there was no other evidence such as eyewitness accounts, the accused was acquitted. When the expert said the body looked as if it had been raped, additional evidence and witnesses were mostly still needed for a conviction. In the one case of incest, a father was acquitted of sexually abusing his daughter even though her hymen was found to be broken. There were no witnesses and no evidence of violence.[33] So, doctors' opinions were important but not overriding. Often, doctors themselves were uncertain about the bodily signs. Sometimes, they differed amongst themselves if multiple experts testified. But nearly always, additional evidence was needed such as stains on bed linen or clothing (indicating intercourse or violence) or statements from eyewitnesses.

Menstruation

Both mother and doctor had types of knowledge that the other did not have. Physicians could use microscopes and examined girls internally, checking for the presence of the hymen. Although they were often unable to establish this conclusively, it was something mothers could and did not examine. On the other hand, mothers were more acquainted with the bodily history and behaviour of their children. Mothers knew if a girl had already had her period and

---

32 NHA, AHA, inv. no. 122, 6 July 1814.
33 NHA, PGNH, inv. no. 223, 16 July 1856. The case file has not been kept and the verdict is very short, it simply mentions that the hymen was torn and there were further traces of violence to the lower body, but it does not mention any physician or examination.

for how long. During trials, they were often asked whether their daughters were menstruating. This seems to have been important to the investigators because a girl who had begun menstruating could be regarded as ready for intercourse and possibly as initiating the intercourse, although this assumption often remained implicit. A man accused of raping his stepdaughter after his wife had died, explained his behaviour by pointing out that the girl had wanted it herself. After all, her periods had started at the age of thirteen which had made her a spinster, which his wife, the girl's mother, had told him.[34]

This opinion seems to have been shared by the medical establishment. In 1863 an eleven-year-old girl, the daughter of a Dutch army major, was raped aboard a ship sailing from the Dutch East Indies, where her father had been stationed, to the Netherlands. The child's mother was asked whether the girl had already had her period. The mother denied this. In addition, the mother was asked if the girl often played with boys. This case revolved around the question whether this girl had been precocious and therefore 'inviting' the sexual assault. Although the ship's doctor didn't think the girl possessed the necessary passions or bodily development for sexual intercourse, and therefore was not 'hysteric', a professor of medicine from the University of Amsterdam was called in, C.B. Tilanus, who testified that, even if of European descent, girls who grew up in the East Indies might develop their passions faster. Nevertheless, Tilanus claimed he did not think this could explain the girl's initiative to sexual intercourse. At the most it could reveal the girl's less powerful resistance and her reticence in telling what had happened.

Interestingly, in this case the father also showed knowledge of his daughter's body. He was present when she was physically examined and testified that she had not become a woman yet.[35] This father was, however, an exception. Generally, knowledge of a girl's body was seen as women's knowledge. This becomes clear from a remark made by neighbouring women in a case involving a fourteen-year-old servant girl, Anna Steltrogge, who had been raped by her master, Evert Bruin, contracting a venereal disease as it turned out later. She had indicated to her mother that she had pain in her lower body. Her mother had recommended rubbing her genitals with bitter almonds and butter milk. The girl had told her master that she felt severe pain and a burning sensation in her lower body caused by a blocked menstruation, in addition to boils in the groins, which made it hard for her to urinate. The master, in his turn, told a neighbour who was a schoolteacher. The schoolteacher advised the girl to see a doctor or apothecary, but the girl refused because it would be too expensive. Therefore he recommended her a medicine: rosemary boiled in milk. After this conversation between the master (the perpetrator) and the schoolteacher, the schoolteacher's wife and (female) servant remarked that they found it very strange that the master knew so much about the girl's body and that it should have been his wife who concerned herself with these female

34   NHA, PGNH, inv. no. 352, 3 July 1867.
35   NHA, PGNH, inv. no. 321, 15 June 1863.

matters. When the schoolteacher's wife, who was partly deaf, asked her husband what his friend had wanted, he responded that his servant girl was about to become a spinster but that 'nature was not working'. His wife understood this, since her own menstruation ('nature') had suddenly stopped when she had fallen in the water at the age of fifteen. Hereupon a doctor had recommended taking rosemary and her period had indeed taken its normal course due to this medicine.[36]

This case is interesting in several respects. Firstly, it shows how knowledge of women's bodies was generally considered to be women's knowledge even though men sometimes interfered. Secondly, it testifies to the presence of early modern notions of the workings of the body. In the early modern period, a common view about shock was that it had bodily effects. This notion can also be found among the lower classes in the Netherlands in the nineteenth century. For instance, a woman's menstruation could suddenly come to a halt when she had been terrified.[37] After a sexual assault, many girls were upset and they were treated for the shock to their nerves. A common treatment was to be bled.[38] Sometimes this was the only treatment and the body was not examined at all. It would be wrong to describe this with the modern notion of trauma because this would imply a separation of body and mind, a notion that didn't exist in the eighteenth and nineteenth centuries. However, it does show that early modern discourses of the body reverberated until the nineteenth century.

Thirdly, the case testifies to lay knowledge of medicine such as the schoolteacher's. Other cases show this as well. For example, physicians and apothecaries recommended washing the genitals with cold water after an assault,[39] but several mothers knew this without the intervention of a doctor.[40] One mother, who was too poor to call in a physician, treated her daughter's swollen genitals with vinegar.[41] In another case, the doctor recommended rubbing the genitals with white wine.[42] In these cases, there doesn't seem to have been a big gap between doctors' and lay people's knowledge of medicine.

Conclusion

To conclude, women were generally regarded as having knowledge of other women's bodies. Partly they had access to this knowledge because they did the laundry, thus possessing a means of social control. Especially mothers were seen as all-knowing in regard to their daughter's bodies and (sexual) be-

36 NHA, AHA, inv. no. 223, 26 July 1819.
37 Duden (1991), p. 69.
38 NHA, AHA, inv. no. 374, 5 July 1826.
39 NHA, PGNH, inv. no. 292, 23 August 1859.
40 NHA, PGNH, inv. no. 323, 2 November 1863.
41 NHA, AHA, inv. no. 353, 1 July 1825.
42 NHA, AHA, inv. no. 397, 1 October 1827.

haviour. Physicians needed this knowledge to do their own examination and report their findings in court. Therefore, to a certain extent this knowledge seems to have been collectively created. This was facilitated by a common discourse on the body and medicine, shared by lay people and physicians. Many early modern notions on the body and medicine continued to exist until the nineteenth century. Men as well as women already knew a lot of medicinal tricks doctors would prescribe them. In this respect it might not be completely accurate to speak of the *transmission* of knowledge, since that would imply a clear point of origin of knowledge that is subsequently disseminated. The sources I have studied would, on the contrary, imply a shared body of knowledge.

However, there were limits to this shared knowledge. I have presented examples of cases in which doctors overruled the knowledge of women. This was made easier when physicians could examine the body in a way mothers could not, for instance by (internally) examining the hymen or by using a microscope to study semen stains on linen. Here, different techniques create different bodies. Therefore, the period I have studied, 1813–1884, seems to be a period in which women and mothers still had a respected knowledge of the female body, a knowledge based on experience not on books. Yet we also see how the professionalization of physicians might detract from this knowledge. In any case, even though their daughters were victims of sexual assault, the agency of mothers in accusing perpetrators, seeking doctors and presenting their own evidence based on experience and knowledge of their daughter's bodies, comes clearly to the fore.

Bibliography

Adelman, Howard Tzvi: Virginity: women's body as a state of mind: destiny becomes biology. In: Diemling, Maria; Veltri, Giuseppe (eds.): The Jewish body. Corporeality, society, and identity in the Renaissance and the early modern period. Leiden; Boston 2009, pp. 179–213.

Alcoff, Linda; Potter, Elizabeth: Introduction: When feminisms intersect epistemology. In: Alcoff, Linda; Potter, Elizabeth (eds.): Feminist epistemologies. London 1993, pp. 1–14.

Bergmann, Carl: Leerboek der medicina forensis voor regtsgeleerden. Utrecht; Amsterdam 1848.

Borg, Helena van der: Vroedvrouwen: beeld en beroep. Ontwikkelingen in het vroedvrouwschap in Leiden, Arnhem, 's-Hertogenbosch en Leeuwarden, 1650–1865. Diss. soc. University of Amsterdam 1992.

Broecke, Jacobus C. van den; Broecke, Philippus van den: De uitoefening der geregtelijke geneeskunde in Nederland: hare gebreken, middelen tot herstel derzelve. Utrecht 1845.

Burke, Peter: A social history of knowledge. From Gutenberg to Diderot. Cambridge 2000.

Dalmiya, Vrinda; Alcoff, Linda: Are 'old wives' tales' justified? In: Alcoff, Linda; Potter, Elizabeth (eds.): Feminist epistemologies. London 1993, pp. 217–244.

Duden, Barbara: The woman beneath the skin. A doctor's patients in eighteenth-century Germany. Cambridge 1991.

Gowing, Laura: Common bodies: women, touch and power in seventeenth-century England. New Haven 2003.

Hekman, Susan: Truth and method: Feminist standpoint theory revisited. In: Signs 22 (1997), pp. 341–365.

Jackson, Louise A.: Child sexual abuse in Victorian England. London 2000.

Jordanova, Ludmilla: The social construction of medical knowledge. In: Social History of Medicine 7 (1995), no. 3, pp. 361–381.

Koster, Wilhelmus A.: Leerboek der gerechtelijke geneeskunde voor artsen en rechtsgeleerden. 2nd edition. Tiel 1877.

Meersch Bosch, Michael van der: Handleiding tot de gerechtelijke geneeskunde. Amsterdam 1814.

Mol, Annemarie: The body multiple: ontology in medical practice. Durham; London 2002.

Mooij, Annet: Geslachtsziekten en besmettingsangst. Een historisch-sociologische studie 1850–1990. Amsterdam 1993.

Porter, Roy: Lay medical knowledge in the eighteenth century: the evidence of the gentleman's magazine. In: Medical History 29 (1985), pp. 138–168.

Porter, Roy: The patient's view: Doing medical history from below. In: Theory and Society 14 (1985), pp. 175–198.

Porter, Roy; Hall, Lesley: The facts of life. The creation of sexual knowledge in Britain, 1650–1950. New Haven; London 1995.

Potter, Elizabeth: Gender and epistemic negotiation. In: Alcoff, Linda; Potter, Elizabeth (eds.): Feminist epistemologies. London 1993, pp. 161–186.

Robertson, Stephen: Crimes against children. Sexual violence and legal culture in New York City, 1880–1960. Chapel Hill; London 2005.

Smith, Pamela H.; Schmidt, Benjamin: Introduction. Knowledge and its making in early modern Europe. In: Smith, Pamela H.; Schmidt, Benjamin (eds.): Making knowledge in early modern Europe. Practices, objects, and texts, 1400–1800. Chicago; London 2007, pp. 1–16.

Stolberg, Michael: Homo patiens: Krankheits- und Körpererfahrung in der frühen Neuzeit. Cologne et al 2003.

Theriot, Nancy M.: Negotiating illness: Doctors, patients and families in the nineteenth century. In: Journal of the History of the Behavioral Sciences 37 (2001), no. 4, pp. 349–368.

Walker, Garthine: Rereading rape and sexual violence in early modern England. In: Gender and History 10 (1998), no. 1, pp. 1–25.

Willems, Dick: Susan's breathlessness – The construction of professionals and laypersons. In: Lachmund, Jens; Stollberg, Gunnar (eds.): The social construction of illness. Illness and medical knowledge in past and present. Stuttgart 1992, pp. 105–114.

Dental care as daily routine: popularization and practice of prophylactic dental hygiene in the German-speaking world, c. 1890–1930[1]

Susanne Hoffmann

Introduction

Today virtually everybody brushes their teeth at least once a day. According to a representative study in Germany (data from 2005), approximately eleven per cent of adults brush their teeth thrice daily, 73 per cent twice daily, and 14 per cent at least once a day.[2] Of the adults 77 per cent use a conventional toothbrush, 38 per cent an electronic toothbrush, 95 per cent toothpaste, and 44 per cent dental floss.[3] At the same time roughly 76 per cent of adults see their dentist regularly for prophylactic reasons, 23 per cent solely if they suffer from acute disorders.[4] Prophylactic dental care thus has obviously become the daily routine. About one hundred years ago this development was by no means foreseeable. The German-speaking world did not experience a massive public campaign to popularize oral hygiene until the last decade of the nineteenth and the first decades of the twentieth century based on new developments in bacteriology, as I will explain in more detail later. This health campaign was part of a much more comprehensive development for which the term "medicalization" is used now. In the social history of medicine it has become habitual to think of medicalization not as a one-way, "top-down" process, from medical professionals to society, but rather as a two-sided process, both "top-down" and "bottom-up", but power relations naturally do interfere with such processes.[5] The historian Francisca Loetz (1993) therefore spoke of the "reciprocal exercise of influence, in which all relevant parties, the state, various kinds of healers and their patients, fight for what is, in their opinion, the best medical treatment".[6]

Transferring Loetz' rather complex model of "medicalization" (she literally speaks of "Medizinische Vergesellschaftung" or "Medical socialization") by analogy to healthcare in general and hygiene in particular, I will argue in the following that the practical appropriation of a "prophylactic style of dental care" was accompanied by severe struggles, above all between pupils and their parents. The process was moderated in social as well as spatial terms. In

1   The research for this contribution was generously supported by a grant of the Robert Bosch Stiftung in Stuttgart (Germany).
2   Micheelis/Reiter (2006), p. 380.
3   Micheelis/Reiter (2006), p. 382.
4   Micheelis/Reiter (2006), p. 385.
5   Cf. Eckart/Jütte (2007), pp. 312–318.
6   Loetz (1993), p. 314.

the first part I will briefly outline the idea of prophylactic dental hygiene in the eighteenth and nineteenth century, under the influence of emerging bacteriology. Secondly, I will look more closely into the subsequent popularization of dental prophylaxis via print media and marketing, hygiene exhibitions and action weeks, and above all school dentistry and school hygiene. Finally, I will turn to dental practice in families, as I will look at the fights about dental care between pupils and their parents at the beginning of the century. Due to my sources, my article focuses on the German-speaking world, i.e. Germany, Austria and Switzerland, in the last decade of the nineteenth and the first third of the twentieth century, that is c. 1890–1930.

Sources and methods

Like the history of medicine in general, the historiography of dentistry has, in the majority of cases, been based up to now on the professional or normative discourses and practices that appear in specific medical journals, in files of dental associations or medical institutions.[7] These sources provide, first of all, valuable insights into the physicians' point of view, their idea of dental prophylaxis and, in the best case, into the dental patient's behaviour. For historians with specific interest in the patient's point of view popular advice literature seems to be more instructive. Although prescriptive advice texts were mostly written by professionals such as medical doctors or dentists, they were addressed at the general public. Besides several monographs on the subject matter, the present paper draws on the third (1874–1878) and sixth (1902–1909) edition of "Meyers Konversations=Lexikon", a German encyclopaedia of general knowledge. In addition, several periodicals of the time that addressed both the elite and the working classes, were systematically analyzed for the present contribution: *Die Gartenlaube*, a rather bourgeois journal of general interest (published 1853–1937), *Vorwärts: Berliner Volksblatt. Zentralorgan der sozialdemokratischen Partei Deutschlands*, a newspaper for members of the social democratic party (published daily 1891–1933), the communist newspaper *Die Rote Fahne* (published 1918–1933), and *Der Naturarzt*, a popular journal for naturopathy (published intermittently since 1862). Beyond that, a few scientific journals which were written for a professional audience, such as *Blätter für Volksgesundheitspflege* (published 1900–1933) and *Die Schulzahnpflege* (published intermittently 1910/11–1936), are informative with regard to our questions, as they offer valuable information on the strategies of professionals to popularize their ideas of oral hygiene.

Concerning practices of personal hygiene, personal documents such as autobiographies, letters or diaries are better suited sources, because they offer insights into the adoption – or rejection – of the aforementioned normative and prescriptive discourses. Therefore the present paper draws on "popular"

---

7   Cf. for instance Hoffmann-Axthelm (1985); Groß (1994); Groß (2006).

autobiographies written by non-famous or amateur authors. All ego-documents mentioned below are part of a larger sample consisting of 155 autobiographies that I analyzed for my doctoral thesis; from this sample I selected seven texts containing comparatively detailed reports on dental hygiene. None of these autobiographies has been published so far. Most texts were written in the last third of the twentieth century, with the authors aiming at circulation inside their families or among the general public. Men and women of all social strata and the birth cohorts from 1890 to 1940 are equally represented in this sample.[8]

Methodologically, I interpreted the named sources within the framework of a discourse analytical approach, extended to include both action theory and sociology of knowledge.[9]

Dental prophylaxis, beauty, and the rise of bacteriology

That oral hygiene was important to maintain a healthy and complete denture, a pleasing face up to a ripe old age, and thus to stay in good health in general, was by no means an authentic invention of late nineteenth century dentistry which had come under the influence of the emerging bacteriology. In fact, the link between dental prophylaxis and beauty is very old and reaches back far into the pre-bacteriological era. The historian Georges Vigarello (1988) argued convincingly that beauty, not health, was central to most personal hygiene practices from the middle ages right up to the eighteenth century.[10] A good example that Vigarello's general observation also applies to oral hygiene is contained in Etienne Bourdet's "Leichte Mittel, den Mund rein und die Zähne gesund zu erhalten" (French orig. 1759, German transl. 1762), a handbook on dental hygiene. Commenting on the relevance of his own treatise, Bourdet opened the foreword with the general assertion that "teeth" were firstly "a natural adornment intrinsically tied to beauty" and only secondly that teeth were "the first tool of our maintenance".[11]

In the nineteenth and early twentieth century, beauty was still an eminently important motive for dental care in both men and women.[12] Despite their vigorous propaganda, dentists complained about people's apparent neglect of health aspects. Karl Röse for instance, a popular representative of the

---

8   The autobiographies originate from the following institutions: Dokumentation lebensgeschichtlicher Aufzeichnungen an der Universität Wien (Doku Wien), Deutsches Tagebucharchiv in Emmendingen (Dta Em), Ludwig-Uhland-Institut für Empirische Kulturwissenschaft an der Universität Tübingen (Lui Tü) und Institut für Populäre Kulturen an der Universität Zürich (Ipk Zh). The authors' family names have been anonymized to protect personal rights as much as possible.
9   Cf. Sarasin (2003).
10 Vigarello (1988), pp. 45–48, 136–137. For Germany analogical Sander (2005), pp. 54–61.
11 Bourdet (1762), p. 3.
12 On aesthetic ideals in general cf. Thoms (1995).

profession in the German "Kaiserreich", elaborated on this point in his essay "On hygiene and cosmetics of teeth" which was published 1893 in the *Deutsche Revue*, a liberal journal. Röse held that the majority of the German population exclusively cared for their teeth because among all "civilized peoples healthy, strong teeth" were seen as "a special adornment".[13] The dentist's assumption was obviously not totally wrong as facial aesthetics turned out to be an important aspect in nineteenth-century German private letters that the historian Nicole Schweig (2009) recently analyzed on a large scale. Some of her young male correspondents were in fact ashamed of their rotten denture in which they saw both an aesthetic and a functional deficiency.[14]

Eighteenth century authors of medical advice literature had already recommended oral prophylaxis. But in contrast to later bacteriological dentistry they had argued within the general framework of dietetics.[15] The above-cited French dentist Etienne Bourdet, for instance, had recommended the following measures to his readers in chapter two of his "Leichte Mittel": remove phlegm every morning, remove leftovers after every meal, eat little sugar, break no hard items with teeth, drink no hot liquids, be careful when changing from warm to cold air, generally keep an orderly lifestyle, treat scurvy and gastrointestinal diseases properly, have venesection when suffering from plethora, regularly see a dentist. In addition, women were asked to stimulate lactation in childbed and have venesection or purging after menopause.[16] Bourdet, whose works saw several editions and were translated into German and many other languages, thus still explained decline in teeth in mechano-chemical terms when he spoke of phlegm, leftovers, sugar, hard items, or hot liquids. Beyond that, he imbedded the function of oral hygiene into a much more comprehensive dietetic regimen, keeping in mind the human body in general and the lifestyle, the "proper life". These kinds of instructions were widely known until well into the second half of the nineteenth century. Contemporaries also spoke of "dental dietetics". The third edition of "Meyers Konversations=Lexikon", a popular German encyclopaedia of general knowledge which was published between 1874 and 1878, still contained similar advice for prophylactic dental health care, but not at such length. What was quite new in nineteenth century advice literature was that toothbrushes were recommended for everybody. The author of the entry "diseases of the teeth and care of the teeth" in "Meyers Konversations=Lexikon" suggested, for instance, to brush in the morning after getting up and in the evening before going to bed, for thorough cleansing of the oral cavity.[17] Bourdet, by comparison, had earlier just spoken of applying a tongue cleaner, tooth picks, sponges, and unspecified "roots" as neces-

---

13   Röse (1893), p. 310.
14   Schweig (2009), p. 163.
15   Cf. Hoffmann-Axthelm (1985), p. 360.
16   Bourdet (1762), pp. 13–19.
17   Meyers Konversations=Lexikon (1874–1878), vol. 15, p. 949. Cf. earlier the entry "tooth powder" in Krünitz (1773–1858), vol. 240, pp. 560–561.

sary devices.[18] One further difference concerned the interval in which care products were to be used: Whereas Bourdet recommended "tooth powder", that is tooth paste, only every 20 to 30 days, Meyer's encyclopaedia, which was written in the 1870s, already propagated its daily use.[19] Dietetic advice literature, such as Etienne Bourdet's above-cited work "Leichte Mittel", was, however, usually addressed at the upper classes, above all at aristocratic and bourgeois men.[20]

The rise of bacteriology fundamentally altered the medical understanding of dental health in the 1880s. In "Die Mikroorganismen der Mundhöhle" (1889) the American dentist Willoughby Dayton Miller, then practising in Berlin, had launched the parasitic-chemical theory of oral cavity health with main features that are still valid today. In both the decalcification of adamantine and the subsequent decomposition of adamantine through germs interacting with carbohydrate sediments from foodstuff, Miller saw the ultimate reason for dental vitiation or caries respectively.[21] Besides the new aetiology of bacteriology, the dentist's instructions for prophylactic dental care remained basically the same. In the sixth edition of "Meyers großes Konversations=Lexikon" (published 1902–1909) the first rule for dental hygiene was still "scrupulous cleanliness". The reader was recommended to use a toothbrush with warm water, dental powder made of soda or soap, and a toothpick if necessary to "[remove] remnants, especially carbohydrates, which easily build acids dissolving the phosphorous and acidic calcium carbonate of teeth". This was considered necessary as "numerous bacteria und funguses that were always present in the mouth, contributed additionally to the decay of teeth", the author explained to his lay audience. Beyond that, he recommended one (for adults) or two (for children) prophylactic checkups a year by a dentist, based on the general value of conservative dentistry. "The earlier a morbid tooth was treated the more easily it was preserved and the lower the danger of healthy teeth becoming affected by their neighbour", the unidentified author argued.[22] Compared to the third edition of "Meyers Konversations=Lexikon", which had been written roughly 30 years earlier, the scientific rationale had indeed changed in the sixth edition, but the strategic approach towards prophylactic or "rational"[23] dental care, as dentists then called it, remained basically unaffected. What had changed in the last decade of the nineteenth and the first third of the twentieth century was only the vig-

---

18 Bourdet (1762), pp. 40–50. Türp (1990) uses the term tooth sweeps ("Zahnfegen") in his ethno-medical comparison for roots which are used to the present day in developing countries for dental hygiene.

19 Bourdet (1762), p. 43; Meyers Konversations=Lexikon (1874–1878), vol. 15, p. 949. On the history of tooth paste cf. Bennion (1988), pp. 146–149; Scholz (1991), pp. 141–147. On the rise of beauty products in general Brede (2005).

20 Cf. Sarasin (2001), pp. 158–162.

21 Hoffmann-Axthelm (1985), pp. 458–462.

22 Meyers großes Konversations=Lexikon (1902–1909), vol. 20, p. 842.

23 Faber (1863), for instance, published a popular handbook under the title "Anleitung zur rationellen Pflege der Zähne und des Mundes".

our with which health professionals now communicated the new bacteriologically founded "prophylactic style of dental care" to the German public.

Popularizing "rational" dental care

The public campaign for "rational" dental care in the outgoing nineteenth and beginning twentieth century was part of a much broader movement that aimed to educate people and was called "Hygienische Volksbelehrung" ("Public Hygiene Instruction"). Medical doctors, officers, and various organizations, members of the affluent bourgeoisie so to speak, were among the most active promoters of a healthy lifestyle which was entirely based on a modern scientific rationale. The movement was particularly active before World War I and again in the 1920s.[24] Next to dental hygiene, personal hygiene in general, venereal diseases, tuberculosis, alcoholism, baby care, food, and living quarters were other key aspects of the movement's activities.[25] Public lectures, personal advice, brochures, posters, films, plays, exhibitions, and (from the mid-1920s onwards) specific health weeks were among the most prominent instruments for the popularization of personal hygiene, as the German ethnographer Gunter Schaible stated (1999).[26]

In fact, contemporaries had the impression that caries had "progressively" risen in the second half of nineteenth century. A Dr Kümmel from Berlin, who represents numerous other authors, wrote in 1903 in the *Archiv für Sozialwissenschaft und Sozialpolitik* about "the continually rising dental decay and its severe consequences" in the previous 30 years.[27] Based on a wide range of statistics on physical examinations in schools and among military recruits Kümmel estimated that just ten per cent of German people had perfectly healthy teeth at the time.[28] Given this data, not only the state of health of the individual person but also of the people had been severely affected by caries, which for Kümmel constituted a "Volkskrankheit". Agitatedly, he argued that both the national military power and the overall performance of the German people were adversely and alarmingly affected by widespread poor dental hygiene.[29] Thus politics eventually also explained the specific efforts to popularize dental prophylaxis.

In terms of oral hygiene, the print media and marketing, exhibitions and action weeks, and – in particular – school hygiene and school dentistry were crucial means within the campaign for "rational" dental care. In what follows, I will take a closer look at those specific tools.

24 Schaible (1999), pp. 82–86. Cf. also Frevert (1985); Labisch (1992), pp. 158–163.
25 Schaible (1999), p. 92.
26 Schaible (1999), pp. 92–93.
27 Kümmel (1903), p. 591.
28 Kümmel (1903), p. 602.
29 Kümmel (1903), p. 597.

Print media and marketing

Mass media experienced a tremendous boom in the "Kaiserreich".[30] Thus edited articles as well as commercial advertisements on personal and dental hygiene could reach an ever growing audience. Both the specifically health-oriented periodicals and the more general periodicals reported on prophylactic dental care on a massive scale after 1900. The *Blätter für Volksgesundheitspflege*, a journal for the general public that was edited by two associations for sanitary instruction, the "Landesausschuss für Hygienische Volksbelehrung in Preußen" and the "Deutscher Verein für Volkshygiene" in cooperation with the "Reichsausschuss" and the "Landesausschüsse für Hygienische Volksbelehrung" between 1900 and 1933, published eight full-length articles on the general subject of oral hygiene[31], twelve shorter contributions[32], and at least four book reviews[33] for the named period: "On dental care" (1901), "On tooth decay" (1902), "On dental care" (1903), "On using a tooth pick" (1905), "Dental hygiene und school dentistry" (1908), "Tooth decay and its prevention" (1911), "The Significance of dental disease for national health", and "General guidelines for dental care" (both 1913) were the headlines of the articles published. Our theme thus reached its climax in the *Blätter für Volksgesundheitspflege* in the decade leading up to World War I (volumes 1901–1913). After that coverage ceased entirely.

The same periodization applies to *Die Gartenlaube*, an "Illustriertes Familienblatt", i.e. a magazine primarily addressed to a general bourgeois readership. *Die Gartenlaube* was published between 1853 and 1937 after which the publication was discontinued.[34] In the two decades leading up to World War I four longer articles were released[35]: "Throat and Mouth Hygiene" (1896), "Alleged teething problems in children" (1899), "An important chapter of dental treatment" (1906), and "False diet and tooth decay" (1912). That was the last article on dental hygiene.

Finally, a systematic content analysis of *Der Naturarzt*[36], a bimonthly journal, that is directed at members of the general public with an interest in

---

30 Wilke (2008), p. 258.

31 *Blätter für Volksgesundheitspflege* 1 (1900/01), pp. 33–36, 49–52; 2 (1902), pp. 213–214; 3 (1903), pp. 165–169; 5 (1905), pp. 343–344; 8 (1908), pp. 107–110; 11 (1911), pp. 132–133; 13 (1913), pp. 49–54, 257–258.

32 *Blätter für Volksgesundheitspflege* 2 (1902), pp. 14, 28–29; 4 (1904), pp. 251–252, 297–298; 5 (1905), pp. 126, 217, 237, 287, 364–365; 6 (1906), pp. 214–215, 218; 7 (1907), p. 46.

33 *Blätter für Volksgesundheitspflege* 1 (1900/01), pp. 124–125; 6 (1906), p. 116; 12 (1912), p. 285.

34 Cf. Ko (2008), pp. 49–111. According to Wilke (2008), p. 276, in 1878 224,000 copies of *Die Gartenlaube* were printed, with a downward tendency though.

35 *Die Gartenlaube* 43 (1896), pp. 680–683; 46 (1899), pp. 268–270; 53 (1906), pp. 429–430; 59 (1912), p. 530. But cf. Ko (2008), p. 133. Based on qualitative data Ko, however, assumes that dental hygiene had been an important subject matter in *Die Gartenlaube* before 1900.

36 *Der Naturarzt* had been the central medium of the naturopathy movement. In 1906 for instance 140,000 copies were printed. Cf. Merta (2003), p. 72.

naturopathy and has been published since 1862 to the present day (intermittently), confirms the pattern just mentioned of the popularization of "rational"
dental care: Between 1894 and 1913 alone, five articles dealt with oral hygiene[37]. After that, coverage was eventually also discontinued.

The message extracted from the aforementioned discourse in the print
medias was generally the same. Everybody must start practising "rational"
prophylactic dental health care, the various authors argued, because dental
health was highly important for both the individual and the people's health
and above all for the beauty of men and women of all ages. This appeal was
printed repeatedly and ended in an extraordinarily high degree of redundancy
in popular instruction.

Propaganda for oral prophylaxis in that time was of course not limited to
the edited content of print media. Dental care and relevant hygiene products
were also central to the marketing campaigns that increasingly flooded Germany from the 1890s onwards. Especially in cities, advertising columns and
posters began to enter public space. Although it was by no means alone, the
growing personal hygiene industry was among the first to market its products,
primarily tooth pastes and mouth washes, on a large scale.[38] Their activities
were part of the rising consumer society.[39] Using again the rather bourgeois
magazine *Die Gartenlaube* as a criterion for mass marketing, the first small advertisement for the mouth wash "Odonta" was published as early as 1897.[40]
Subsequently, since 1899 the tooth paste "Kalodont" was being promoted to
the readership[41]; it was the first tooth paste sold in a tube[42]. The first adverts
for the anti-bacterial mouth wash "Odol", whose brand name and design are
still well known today, appeared from 1907 onwards in *Die Gartenlaube*.[43]
"Odol" was manufactured by a clever businessman from Dresden, Karl August Lingner. He was also one of the most active promoters of the "Hygienische Volksbelehrung" movement, of the Dresden hygiene exhibition in
1911 as well as the later "Deutsches Hygiene Museum".[44] Lingner's biography
illustrates how philanthropic and commercial interests, editorial and marketing campaigns in print media complemented each other in the overall goal of
promoting "rational" dental care.

With regard to the social aspects of (assumed) personal hygiene practices,
it is instructive to compare the advertising sections in *Die Gartenlaube* with
newspapers typically addressed to a working class audience. For one, the jour-

---

37 *Der Naturarzt* 22 (1894), pp. 193–213; 35 (1907), pp. 31–33, 37–38; 36 (1908), pp. 29–33,
    52–53, 299–300; 37 (1909), pp. 47–49; 41 (1913), p. 107. The next article on dental care
    appeared 16 years later in *Der Naturarzt* 57 (1929), pp. 252–255.
38 For general information on the rise of marketing cf. Reinhardt (1993); on marketing of
    personal hygiene products Thoms (2009).
39 Cf. last Trentmann (2009).
40 *Die Gartenlaube* 44 (1897), no. 1.
41 *Die Gartenlaube* 46 (1899), no. 2.
42 Cf. Scholz (1991), pp. 153–154; Seidel (2002), p. 39.
43 *Die Gartenlaube* 54 (1907), no. 2.
44 Hodgson (1993).

nal *Vorwärts*, which was directed at members of the social democratic party[45], contained no single advertisement for prophylactic products for the oral cavity (such as toothpaste, toothbrush or mouth wash) between 1891 and 1924, whereas various other consumer goods (like clothing or detergents) were routinely advertised. Before 1924, only dentists or other dental practitioners had regularly offered their curative services (such as filling or extracting teeth or prostheses) to anguished potential patients.[46] Among the first advertisements for prophylactic products[47] was the toothpaste "Chlorodont" that the Dresden chemist Ottomar Heinsenius von Mayenburg had produced serially since 1907/11[48]. The advertisers promoted "Chlorodont" as a remedy for calculus, dental plaque, and bad breath (see figure 2).[49] So besides dental health, considerations of aesthetics and beauty were important buying incentives even in the working class press. "White teeth!", "Unstained teeth" or "2 tips for personal hygiene" were among the promises in an advertisement published in *Die Rote Fahne* (1930), a German communist newspaper.[50] The message spread by the worker's press was therefore by no means different from that broadcast by upper class media, but in the latter, commercial propaganda for dental prophylaxis had set in a quarter of a century earlier.

The comparatively low purchasing power of the lower classes was certainly a crucial factor in the entrepreneurs' longstanding disregard for the working-class press, as the following example illustrates: according to the official pricelist (no. 585) of Lingner's company, a tin tube of "Odol" toothpaste cost 1 Reichsmark (RM) in 1930.[51] Given that the average working class family had a monthly income of 250 RM, dental hygiene products were still more or less luxury goods in the lower classes in that year.[52] It was therefore certainly not a coincidence that the first advertisement for dental prophylaxis published in *Vorwärts* (1924) praised the "reasonably priced toothpaste Novidont".[53]

45 C. 1900 52,000 copies of the *Vorwärts* were published and 1914 160,000 copies. Cf. Wilke (2008), p. 265.
46 Cf. for example *Vorwärts* 8 (1891), no. 8; 17 (1900), no. 5; 27 (1910), no. 1 (see figure 1).
47 Cf. for instance *Vorwärts* 41 (1924); no. 27; 42 (1925), nos. 6, 36, 68.
48 Gubig/Köpcke (1997), pp. 8–11.
49 *Vorwärts* 42 (1925), no. 6.
50 *Die Rote Fahne* 13 (1930), nos. 20, 25, 181.
51 Deutsches Hygiene Museum Dresden, 2010/110.
52 The example is taken from Hagemann (1990), pp. 32–33, based on a book of household accounts of a gardener family of six persons. From their average monthly income of 252 RM the family spent only 2,70 RM, that is 1,1 per cent, on cleansing materials and personal hygiene. With 157,50 RM or 62,5 per cent the greatest part of their income was spent on food, drinks, tobacco, gas, and electricity.
53 *Vorwärts* 41 (1924), no. 27.

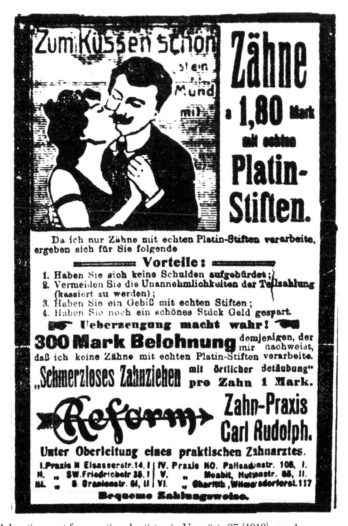

Figure 1: Advertisement for curative dentistry in Vorwärts 27 (1910), no. 1

Die drei Schönheitsfehler des Mundes

1. Der Zahnstein

ist die Absatz des Speichels ähnlich wie der Kesselstein des Wassers. Er hat eine graugrüne, braune bis schwarze Färbung und ist zunächst ein Schönheitsfehler, der den Zähnen ein häßliches, ungepflegtes Aussehen gibt und einen üblen faulreges Geruch aus dem Munde verursacht. Er ist aber auch ein höchst gefährlicher Feind des Gebisses, weil er Zahnfleisch- und Kieferschwund sowie Zahnfleischentzündungen und Eiterungen verursacht. Er ist äußerst festsitzend und hart oft wie bei einer harten Kruste den ganzen Zahnhals und verursacht ein Lockerwerden der Zähne.

2. Mißfarbener Zahnbelag

hervorgerufen durch starkes Rauchen von Zigarren und Zigaretten, ist weniger schädlich, aber ein um so auffallenderer Schönheitsfehler des Gebisses. Wie entfernt man Zahnstein und Zahnbelag? Weder mit Mundwasser noch mit sogenannten Lösungsmitteln; in dieser Beziehung ähnelt der Zahnstein auch dem Kesselstein, gegen den allerlei Lösungsmittel sich als wirkungslos erwiesen haben und die rein mechanische Beseitigung sich am besten bewährt. Millionen, die heute Chlorodont täglich in Gebrauch haben und ihre schönen weißen Zähne dieser Zahnpflege verdanken, haben es selbst ausprobiert, daß Mundwasser die mechanische Reinigungskraft der mikroskopisch keinen reinen Kreide im Chlorodont nicht ersetzen kann.

3. Übler Mundgeruch

als Folge mangelhafter Zahnpflege macht sich weniger dem davon Betroffenen, als seiner näheren Umgebung bemerkbar. Neutrale Salze im Chlorodont, die eine vermehrte Speichelbildung und dadurch eine natürliche Mundreinigung bewirken, in Verbindung mit dem herrlich erfrischenden Pfefferminzgeschmack beseitigen diesen markanten Schönheitsfehler unmittelbar. Jeder Tube Chlorodont ist eine genaue Gebrauchsanweisung beigefügt. Chlorodont-Zahnpaste und die dafür geeignete Chlorodont-Zahnbürste mit gezahntem Borsten- schnitt sind die besten Hilfsmittel gegen den gefürchteten Zahnstein, mißfarbenen Zahnbelag und den oft damit verbundenen üblen Mundgeruch.

beseitigt Chlorodont-Zahnpaste

Figure 2: One of the advertisements for preventive dental care in Vorwärts 42 (1925), no. 6

Hygiene exhibitions and action weeks

Hygiene exhibitions and local action weeks were important aspects of public hygiene instruction ("Hygienische Volksbelehrung") in the early twentieth century. Although such events had obviously reached a narrower audience than the aforementioned print media, "rational" oral hygiene was still included in the conceptual design of these events. This applies above all to the first "Internationale Hygiene-Ausstellung" of 1911 in Dresden where a collection on the human body ("Der Mensch") was exhibited in the popular hall ("Populäre Halle"). One section of that exhibition was solely devoted to personal health care including dental hygiene. According to the original exhibition catalogue, "tables, pictures, preparations, and extended replications" of tooth diseases were shown as well as means of cure and prevention of such ailments.[54] This approach was necessary, the organizers of the exhibition argued, because "this specific branch of general personal hygiene had by and large been neglected and had only begun to attract attention in the past few years".[55] Later, in the 1920s, the collection "Der Mensch" attracted large crowds when it was exhibited all over the Reich.[56] At the next national health exhibition, the "Große Ausstellung für Gesundheitspflege, soziale Fürsorge und Leibesübungen" (Gesolei) that took place in Düsseldorf in 1926, much space was again given to dentistry and dental hygiene.[57]

In the 1920s, specific dental hygiene exhibitions were even organized on a local level. In the city of Karlsruhe, to give only one example, a "Zahnhygienische Ausstellung" took place from September 5 to 13, 1925. The event started with an open competition for school children, under the heading: "Who has the best looked after teeth?".[58] In Berlin Kreuzberg, to mention another example from the same year, a "dental care week" was organized where pupils were, for one week, instructed in dental care next to their regular lessons.[59] School children had, in fact, emerged as a new focal point in the broad popularization of "rational" dental hygiene.

School hygiene and school dentistry

The expansion of school hygiene was a broader development at the turn of the nineteenth to the twentieth century, when an ever growing number of cities appointed special school doctors who took on the duty of pupil's health care from municipal public health officers.[60] Dental care, with specific school

54 Internationale Hygiene-Ausstellung (1911), p. 49.
55 Internationale Hygiene-Ausstellung (1911), p. 49.
56 Cf. Schaible (1999), pp. 107–109.
57 Kessler (1926); Kessler (1927).
58 Oehrlein (1925), p. 428.
59 *Die Schulzahnpflege* 14 (1926), p. 29.
60 For Prussia see Bennack (1990), pp. 274–278.

dentists being in charge of school dental clinics, had been called for right from the beginning of the school hygiene movement. A German encyclopaedia on school hygiene, the "Enzyklopädisches Handbuch der Schulhygiene" (1904), included emphatic demands for school dentistry. School dentists, the author of the entry "dentist" had argued, must be instrumental in instructing the pupils in prophylactic dental care, in preventing and treating tooth disease.[61] In 1909 the "Deutsches Zentralkomitee für Zahnpflege in den Schulen", a professional organization for the promotion of dental care in schools, was founded; dentists were among the most active promoters.[62] Between 1910/11 and 1936 the "Zentralkomitee" even issued (intermittently) a journal with the title *Die Schulzahnpflege* ("School dental hygiene") (a supplement to *Zahnärztliche Mitteilungen*, a scientific journal for dentists). The medical historian Dominik Groß convincingly argued that the dentists' commitment was in most cases neither based on pure altruism nor philanthropy, but part of the "difficult professionalization" that Germany's dentists underwent at the beginning of the century.[63] Only with the 1914 "Reichsversicherungsordnung" dental treatment became explicitly a service included in Bismarck's compulsory health insurance fund and the monopoly of academically trained dentists.[64] Following the deregulation of the German medical market 1869/72 ("Kurierfreiheit") and until 1952 qualified dentists ("Zahnärzte") were faced with the competition of dental practitioners who were not academically trained ("Dentisten").[65] Only in 1919 German dentists were granted the right to gain doctoral degrees.[66]

The first dental clinic in a school was established in Straßburg (then under German occupation) in October 1902, under the auspices of the dentist Dr Ernst Jessen. The second clinic opened six weeks later in Darmstadt (Hesse).[67] In *Die Schulzahnpflege* of 1929 Dr Hans Joachim Tholuck published the following figures on the spreading of school dental clinics in the German Reich:

Year	Number of school dental clinics
1909	37
1914	81
1925	261
1927	560
1928	653

Table 1: School dental clinics in the German Reich 1909–1928, Tholuck (1929), p. 25

61 Wehmer (1904), pp. 1004–1014.
62 Groß (1994), pp. 309–312.
63 Groß (1994), p. 12.
64 Groß (1994), pp. 257–304.
65 Groß (2006).
66 Groß (1994), p. 248.
67 Groß (1994), pp. 308–309.

According to Tholuck's statistics, school dentistry grew most during the second half of the 1920s, but in rural areas where dentists were generally scarce the provision of school dental clinics often remained unsatisfactory, another dentist argued in the same year.[68]

The majority of school dental clinics in the 1920s were under the auspices of medically trained dentists.[69] Free treatment of the pupils remained a highly controversial topic among school dentists and independent or panel doctors, as both groups were competing with each other for local supremacy and patients.[70] For the present contribution, the introduction of prophylactic dental care practices in schools is crucial. Wall panels displaying the anatomy of teeth, tooth disease and dental care circulated in schools. One of these wall panels, "Die Zähne und ihre Pflege" by the Straßburg dentist Dr Ernst Jessen is shown below (see figure 3). It gives the reader an impression of the core messages this medium could carry. Next to an anatomic model of the maxilla at different ages the wall panel contained 14 short statements on dental care that were simple and easy to remember[71]:

1. At age 2 ½ every child has 20 teeth.
2. At age 6 the first lasting molar appears in the back of the mouth.
3. The change of teeth takes place from 7 to 14 years.
4. At age 12 the second big molars appear, and at age 18 to 40 the wisdom teeth.
5. Healthy teeth are essential for a healthy stomach and general physical health.
6. For children milk teeth are more important than permanent teeth are for adults.
7. Healthy milk teeth are a precondition for healthy permanent teeth.
8. From early childhood teeth must be brushed daily in the morning and especially in the evening.
9. From age 3 onwards yearly dental check-ups are necessary.
10. As soon as there are signs of decay, teeth should be filled before pain occurs.
11. The mouth, as the entrance to our body, must be in complete health.
12. To keep the oral cavity clean all roots that are not suited for inlays must be extracted, dental calculus must be removed regularly.
13. The own teeth must be preserved by inlays in time because artificial teeth are only a makeshift.
14. Good chewing is almost digesting, that's why you must care for your teeth.

In summary it can be said that oral hygiene propaganda in schools strategically aimed both at "rational" dental care and medicalization.

Apart from dentists, ordinary school teachers also instructed their pupils in prophylactic dental care. Professionals occasionally stated in medical journals, that school dentists knew well that they were dependent on the active contributions of school teachers if they wanted to achieve their overall goal of popularizing the new style of dental care.[72] Already in the 1850s, many class

---

68 Hoffmann (1929), p. 517.
69 Hoffmann (1929), p. 517.
70 Groß (1994), pp. 313–316.
71 Jessen/Loos/Schlaeger (1904), p. 32.
72 Hertel (1925); Kientopf (1930).

readers contained information on dental prophylaxis.[73] Since the turn of the century, dental care even had become part of the regular teacher training in Prussia. At least in theory, oral hygiene could therefore be part of natural science or any other subject lessons.[74] The impact of school hygiene and school dentistry on oral hygiene practices in everyday bath room life were certainly striking as I will argue in the following paragraph.

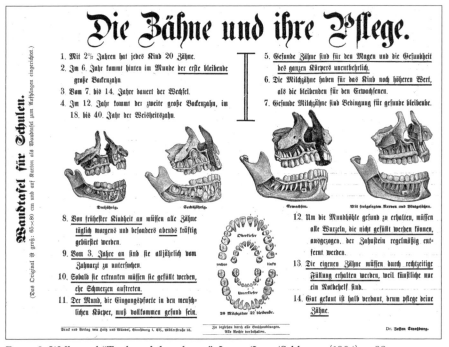

Figure 3: Wall panel "Teeth and dental care", Jessen/Loos/Schlaeger (1904), p. 32

Pupils, parents, and new practices of prophylactic dental care

Although the idea of prophylactic dental care did by no means originate in nineteenth century bacteriologic dentistry, actual dental care practices were mostly unknown to broad parts of society in early modern times and throughout the nineteenth century. It is indeed fair to assume, as the historian Robert Jütte (1996) argues, that caries prevalence was relatively low then due to the generally lower sugar consumption. Toothache was nevertheless a widespread experience.[75] Many ego-documents of that period contain rather elaborate descriptions by early modern sufferers from all social ranks.[76]

---

73   Pöggeler (2000), pp. 160–181.
74   Krei (1995), p. 101.
75   Jütte (1996), p. 39.
76   Jütte (1996), p. 39; Hoffmann (2005), p. 154.

The adoption of dental prophylaxis as a daily routine grew in a socially and spatially differentiated way. The gentry and bourgeoisie were obviously the first to adopt the "prophylactic style of dental health care" in the course of the nineteenth century. The autobiographies of men and women who were born after c. 1890 in that social setting do not contain any sign of conflict between pupils and their parents on the question of proper dental hygiene. A paragraph in Richard S.' (born 1896) autobiography is certainly instructive with regard to the widespread early habituation to prophylactic behaviour patterns in the upper social strata. In memory of his little son (who died 1936 at the age of six) the lawyer and administrative officer proudly wrote "zealously he dedicated himself to body and dental hygiene in the bathroom where we often found long strips of toothpaste squeezed out".[77] And even orthodontics was occasionally and willingly accepted among the gentry and the bourgeoisie as an expression of a modern and scientific dentistry. "As my sister M. had an underbite with her second teeth", Baroness Helene R. (born 1888) explained looking back, "she was taken to a clever dentist who tried to push her teeth back with a machine. It was dangerous for M., but unfortunately she did not benefit from the treatment."[78]

In the lower classes and rural areas the situation turned out to be different. The sample of popular autobiographies, on which the present work is based, contains several indications that a "traditional style of dental care" was indeed widespread around 1900 among the lower classes and in rural areas. One example goes back to Bruno F. (born 1896). The mechanical engineer who grew up in rural Wuerttemberg described the dental care practices in his youth at great length:

> As a schoolboy I suffered already from bad back teeth, we called them M-teeth then. My mother or sister would drip clove drops into my mouth that smelled better than they were helpful, but sooner or later the pain would cease. Nobody thought of seeing a dentist because of that. The next dentist had his surgery in He., our district town. One hour walk to the train station, 90 minutes in a small train, half an hour walk from the train station to the surgery, that is at least three hours in total, on top of that came the waiting time and the fees, that was simply out of the question. Furthermore, my father held the opinion that back teeth were not really important, the main thing was that the visible front and canine teeth were all right.[79]

Looking back at his apprenticeship a Swiss baker (born 1907) retrospectively complained that his mother had put "neither nightdress nor soap nor toothbrush" into his bag when he left home, to give another example of the scant prophylaxis in sub-bourgeois contexts.[80] The last example of poor prophylaxis in my sample comes from Genoveva F. (born 1934). In a handwritten

77 Richard S.: Augenblicksbilder meiner Lebenswanderschaft (Eine dankbare Rückschau auf sieben Jahrzehnte). Doku Wien c. 1967, p. 110.

78 Helene R.: Die Heimatsucherin: Lebensgeschichte einer Stiftsdame im Hradsiner Damenstift; part I–IV a–c. Doku Wien c. 1962–1970, part I, p. 33.

79 Bruno F.: Über neun Jahrzehnte hinweg. Lui Tü c. 1984, p. 194.

80 Mr. "Li der Widder": [Without title]. Ipk Zh 30 c. 1908, p. 29.

appendix to her autobiography the unskilled Austrian farm worker provided an account of how she invested her very first salary, in 1949, in both tooth-brush and toothpaste. Because she knew then that "not many people owned a toothbrush", Genoveva F. explained, she was teased at every opportunity by her immediate surrounding. "You have pretty snow-white teeth today", the others apparently teased her.[81] So, in summary, "traditional" dental care then still meant: no regular prophylactic hygiene, no preventive dentist checkups, no inlays for carious teeth to preserve the denture for as long as possible, but extraction of teeth as soon as they were finally rotten in the mouth, and self-help in the meantime. Given this qualitative evidence, the above-cited nerv-ous scandalization of poor dental hygiene by dentists among wide parts of so-ciety around 1900 was not entirely mistaken and, if anything, it had died out before the first half of the twentieth century had come to an end.

Pupils frequently introduced the "modern" prophylactic practices they learned at school to their lower class and rural families in the first third of the twentieth century. My autobiographic sample provides evidence for at least two severe conflicts between children and parents over the matter of dental care in the period of investigation. One typical example is that of a Swiss woman (born 1910), the daughter of an unskilled worker and caretaker, who in retrospect bitterly blamed her father for having neglected dental prophylaxis: "We children were not allowed to get inlays from a dentist. Father thought that teeth should decay and later be replaced by prostheses." She continued blam-ing the father's backwardness with an example: "Once I had toothache. I had to go to the dentist to get the aching tooth extracted. But the dentist refused to do this. He said that it was a pity and such a tooth should have an inlay. But father insisted. Mother had to go along with me to the dentist for the tooth to be extracted. Later, when I was older, I bitterly regretted it."[82] Some twenty pages later the woman renewed her accusation of wilful neglect of dental care in her family: "When I later had the chance, my neglected teeth had to be treated. Now I had to pay for the fact that nothing had been done to care for them."[83]

It remains an open question whether pupils like the above-cited Swiss woman came into contact with a "prophylactic style of dental care" at school. Unfortunately the analyzed autobiographic sample provides no direct proof for the named way of transmission. Dentists and doctors were, however, the first to frankly discuss in medical journals that a change of personal hygiene routines was a tedious and complex process that would take at least two gen-erations. As early as 1909 the directorate of the "Verein für naturgemäße Ge-sundheitspflege" criticized in its popular journal *Der Naturarzt* that adults at the

81   Genoveva F.: Nur von meinem Mann die Tochter!; part I and II. Doku Wien c. 1993/1999,
     w/o p.
82   Mrs. "Jugenderinnerungen": Meine Jugenderinnerungen. Ipk Zh 12 c. 1980, p. 6.
83   Mrs. "Jugenderinnerungen": Meine Jugenderinnerungen. Ipk Zh 12 c. 1980, pp. 12, 19.
     Cf. also Bruno F.: Über neun Jahrzehnte hinweg. Lui Tü c. 1984, p. 194.

time were "too weak to fight their own vices".[84] And still in 1925 another dentist argued in *Die Schulzahnpflege* that although the family was actually responsible for hygiene education, many parents were not yet able to exercise their duty.[85] Hence school dentists consciously formulated the strategic approach that pupils should educate their parents. Commenting on the high value of a competition for pupils in the context of a local dental hygiene exhibition in Karlsruhe, Dr Oehrlein from Heidelberg for instance explained in the same year that: "the pupils were thus skilfully [...] assigned the task of teaching their parents the importance of dental care and of referring to the exhibition."[86] Five years later, in 1930, professionals were disillusioned regarding the actual potential of school dentistry to bring about change and the factual longevity of "traditional" dental care:

> The awareness, that even the instructions that were introduced together with regular school dental care cannot educate the youth to personal oral and dental hygiene, has gradually reached everybody practicing dental care in school. Like the school doctor the school dentist depends on the support of the schools. One could argue that school is already too late, because education for hygiene must start with infants and is therefore the parents' task. In the light of most parents' attitude to hygiene only the generation that already experienced such an education in young years will teach their children accordingly, and as long as a large part of the population is far away from any kind of hygiene, schools must carry on the work of education.[87]

Yet, in the long run the knowledge transmission from pupils to parents proved to be effective.

Conclusion

Based on a broad range of both prescriptive and autobiographical sources the present contribution reconstructs the process in which a "prophylactic style of dental care" almost became daily routine between the last decade of the nineteenth and over the further course of the twentieth century. The actual struggles that took place in several lower class and rural households on the issue of dental prophylaxis which men as well as women remembered in their autobiographies were taken as proof for my thesis that school dentistry and school hygiene were crucial for both the broad popularization and the subsequent and – most notably – comprehensive appropriation of prophylaxis in all social strata. The depicted implementation of the new bacteriologically based "prophylactic style of dental care" in German daily life drew a rather complex picture of medicalization or hygienization. It goes well with Francisca Loetz' concept of "Medizinische Vergesellschaftung" as the process was moderated socially and spatially and was in itself laden with conflict. Conflicts were car-

84 Finkh-Schleswig (1909), p. 48.
85 Hertel (1925), p. 18.
86 Oehrlein (1925), p. 428.
87 Kientopf (1930), p. 31.

ried out between pupils and their parents who belonged to two successive generations. To change behaviour patterns in a society was therefore a tedious process that took at least half a century. In the end, the medicalization of oral hygiene turned out to be a dual process in which the strategies of medical doctors, clever entrepreneurs, and professionals met the awakening consumer's demand – that was, however, indirectly induced by professionals – not only for medical prevention but also for aesthetics that stimulated the demand for prevention even among the lower classes.

Bibliography

Published sources

Blätter für Volksgesundheitspflege. Gemeinverständliche Zeitung des Landesausschusses für Hygienische Volksbelehrung in Preußen und des Deutschen Vereins für Volkshygiene (1900–1933).

Bourdet, Etienne: Leichte Mittel, den Mund rein und die Zähne gesund zu erhalten. Leipzig 1762.

Der Naturarzt. Zeitschrift des Deutschen Bundes der Vereine für Gesundheitspflege und arzneilose Heilweise (1889–1942).

Die Gartenlaube. Illustriertes Familienblatt (1853–1937).

Die Rote Fahne. Zentralorgan der KPD (Sektion der Kommunistischen Internationalen) (1918–1933).

Die Schulzahnpflege. Zeitschrift des Deutschen Zentralkomitees für Zahnpflege in den Schulen (1910/11–1936).

Faber, Carl-Maria: Anleitung zur rationellen Pflege der Zähne und des Mundes. Wien 1863.

Finckh-Schleswig, K.: Wie unser Verein die Zahnpflege fördert. In: Der Naturarzt 37 (1909), pp. 47–49.

Hertel, E.: Ueber Unterricht in Zahnpflege. In: Die Schulzahnpflege 13 (1925), pp. 17–19.

Hoffmann, K.F.: Ueber den gegenwärtigen Stand der Schulzahnpflege, der zahnärztlichen Krankenkassen-Kliniken, der zahnärztlichen Stationen in Krankenhäusern sowie einer Statistik über die zahnärztlich ungenügend versorgten Orte in Deutschland. In: Zahnärztliche Mitteilungen 20 (1929), pp. 516–519.

Internationale Hygiene-Ausstellung. Offizieller Führer durch die Internationale Hygiene-Ausstellung Dresden 1911 und durch Dresden und Umgebung. Berlin 1911.

Jessen, Ernst; Loos, Otto; Schlaeger: Zahnhygiene in Schule und Heer. Straßburg 1904.

Kessler, Wilhelm: Zahn-, Mund- und Kieferheilkunde auf der Gesolei. In: Zahnärztliche Mitteilungen 17 (1926), pp. 449–452.

Kessler, Wilhelm: Die Schulzahnpflege auf der Gesolei. In: Die Schulzahnpflege 15 (1927), pp. 57–58.

Kientopf, J.: Zur Frage der hygienischen Erziehung in der Schule. In: Die Schulzahnpflege 18 (1930), pp. 31–34.

Krünitz, Johann Georg: Oekonomische Encyclopädie, oder allgemeines System der Staats= Stadt= Haus= und Landwirthschaft. In alphabetischer Ordnung. 242 vols. Berlin 1773–1858.

Kümmel, H.: Die progressive Zahncaries in Schule und Heer und die zahnhygienischen Aufgaben der Sanitätsbehörden im Interesse der Volkswirtschaft. In: Archiv für Sozialwissenschaft und Sozialpolitik 18 (1903), pp. 591–630.

Meyers großes Konversations=Lexikon. Ein Nachschlagewerk des allgemeinen Wissens. 6th ed. 21 vols. Leipzig; Wien 1902–1909.

Meyers Konversations=Lexikon. Eine Encyclopädie des allgemeinen Wissens. 3rd ed. 16 vols. Leipzig 1874–1878.

Oehrlein: Die "Zahnhygienische" Ausstellung in Karlsruhe. In: Die Schulzahnpflege 13 (1925), p. 428.

Röse, Karl: Über die Hygiene und Kosmetik der Zähne. In: Deutsche Revue über das gesamte nationale Leben der Gegenwart 18 (1893), pp. 309–329.

Tholuck, Hans Joachim: Der augenblickliche Stand der Schulzahnpflege im Deutschen Reiche. In: Die Schulzahnpflege 17 (1929), pp. 25–27.

Vorwärts. Berliner Volksblatt; Zentralorgan der Sozialdemokratischen Partei Deutschlands (1891–1933).

Wehmer, Richard (ed.): Enzyklopädisches Handbuch der Schulhygiene. Wien; Leipzig 1904.

Literature

Bennack, Jürgen: Gesundheit und Schule. Zur Geschichte der Hygiene im preußischen Volksschulwesen. Köln; Weimar; Wien 1990.

Bennion, Elisabeth: Alte zahnärztliche Instrumente. Ed. by Marielene Putscher and Ulrich Lohse. Köln 1988.

Brede, Christina: Das Instrument der Sauberkeit: Die Entwicklung der Massenproduktion von Feinseifen in Deutschland 1850 bis 2000. Münster et al 2005.

Eckart, Wolfgang; Jütte, Robert: Medizingeschichte. Eine Einführung. Köln; Weimar; Wien 2007.

Frevert, Ute: "Fürsorgliche Belagerung". Hygienebewegung und Arbeiterfrauen im 19. und frühen 20. Jahrhundert. In: Geschichte und Gesellschaft 11 (1985), pp. 420–446.

Groß, Dominik: Die schwierige Professionalisierung der deutschen Zahnärzteschaft (1867–1919). (= Europäische Hochschulschriften, Reihe III, no. 609) Frankfurt/Main et al 1994.

Groß, Dominik: Vom "Gebißarbeiter" zum "staatlich geprüften Dentisten": Der Berufsbildungsprozess der nichtapprobierten Zahnbehandler (1869–1952). In: Groß, Dominik: Beiträge zur Geschichte und Ethik der Zahnheilkunde. Würzburg 2006, pp. 99–125.

Gubig, Thomas; Köpcke, Sebastian: Chlorodont. Biographie eines Markenproduktes. Dresden 1997.

Hagemann, Karen: Frauenalltag und Männerpolitik. Alltagsleben und gesellschaftliches Handeln von Arbeiterfrauen in der Weimarer Republik. Bonn 1990.

Hodgson, Anne: Von der Gartenlaube zum Großbetrieb. Die Odol-Geschichte. In: Roth, Martin; Scheske, Manfred; Täubrich, Hans-Christian (eds.): In aller Munde: Einhundert Jahre Odol. Stuttgart 1993, pp. 31–49.

Hoffmann, Susanne: Gesundheit und Krankheit bei Ulrich Bräker (1735–1798). (= Zürcher Medizingeschichtliche Abhandlungen 297) Dietikon 2005.

Hoffmann-Axthelm, Walter: Die Geschichte der Zahnheilkunde. Berlin 1985.

Jütte, Robert: "La douleur des dents est la plus grande": Zur Geschichte des Zahnschmerzes in der Frühen Neuzeit. In: Medizin, Gesellschaft und Geschichte 18 (1996), pp. 37–54.

Ko, Jae-Baeck: Wissenschaftspopularisierung und Frauenberuf. Diskurs um Gesundheit, hygienische Familie und Frauenrolle im Spiegel der Familienzeitschrift Die Gartenlaube in der zweiten Hälfte des 19. Jahrhunderts. (= Europäische Hochschulschriften, Reihe III, no. 1052) Frankfurt/Main et al 2008.

Krei, Thomas: Gesundheit und Hygiene in der Lehrerbildung: Strukturen und Prozesse im Rheinland seit 1870. Köln; Weimar; Wien 1995.

Labisch, Alfons: Homo Hygienicus. Gesundheit und Medizin in der Neuzeit. Frankfurt/Main 1992.

Loetz, Francisca: Vom Kranken zum Patienten. "Medikalisierung" und medizinische Verge-
    sellschaftung am Beispiel Badens 1750–1850. Stuttgart 1993.
Merta, Sabine: Wege und Irrwege zum modernen Schlankheitskult. Diätkost und Körperkul-
    tur als Suche nach neuen Lebensstilformen 1880–1930. (= Studien zur Geschichte des All-
    tags 22) Stuttgart 2003.
Micheelis, Wolfgang; Reiter, Florian: Soziodemographische und verhaltensbezogene Aspekte
    oraler Risikofaktoren in den vier Alterskohorten. In: Micheelis, Wolfgang; Schiffer, Ulrich
    (eds.): Vierte Deutsche Mundgesundheitsstudie (DM IV). Köln 2006, pp. 375–398.
Pöggeler, Ansgar: Zahnmedizin und Schule im Spiegel von Lehrer- und Schülerbüchern
    zwischen 1800 und 1950. (= Studien zur Pädagogik, Andragogik und Gerontagogik 48)
    Frankfurt/Main et al 2000.
Reinhardt, Dirk: Von der Reklame zum Marketing. Geschichte der Wirtschaftswerbung in
    Deutschland. Berlin 1993.
Sander, Sabine: Die dreißig Schönheiten der Frau – Ärztliche Ratgeber der Frühen Neuzeit.
    In: Stahnisch, Frank; Steger, Florian (eds.): Medizin, Geschichte und Geschlecht. Körper-
    historische Rekonstruktionen von Identitäten und Differenzen. (= Geschichte und Philoso-
    phie der Medizin 1) Stuttgart 2005, pp. 41–62.
Sarasin, Philipp: Reizbare Maschinen. Eine Geschichte des Körpers 1765–1914. Frankfurt/
    Main 2001.
Sarasin, Philipp: Geschichtswissenschaft und Diskursanalyse. Frankfurt/Main 2003.
Schaible, Gunter: Sozial- und Hygiene-Ausstellungen. Objektpräsentation im Industriali-
    sierungsprozess. Diss. phil. Tübingen 1999.
Scholz, Joachim Dieter: Die Geschichte der Zahnpaste. Diss. med. Bonn 1991.
Schweig, Nicole: Gesundheitsverhalten von Männern: Gesundheit und Krankheit in Briefen,
    1800–1950. (= Medizin, Gesellschaft und Geschichte, Beiheft 33) Stuttgart 2009.
Seidel, Brigitte: Maggi, Odol, Persil & Co. erobern den ländlichen Haushalt. Husum 2002.
Thoms, Ulrike: Dünn und dick, schön und häßlich. Schönheitsideal und Körpersilhouette in
    der Werbung 1850–1950. In: Borscheid, Peter; Wischermann, Clemens (eds.): Bilder des
    Alltags. Werbung in der Konsumgesellschaft des 19. und 20. Jahrhunderts; Festschrift für
    Jürgen Teuteberg. (= Studien zur Geschichte des Alltags 13) Stuttgart 1995, pp. 242–281.
Thoms, Ulrike: Körper, Kultur, Konsum: Die Konsumgeschichte alltäglicher Hygiene. In:
    Haupt, Heinz-Gerhard; Torp, Claudius (eds.): Die Konsumgesellschaft in Deutschland
    1890–1990. Frankfurt/Main 2009, pp. 97–113.
Trentmann, Frank: The long history of consumer society: Chronologies, practices, and poli-
    tics in Modern Europe. In: Archiv für Sozialgeschichte 49 (2009), pp. 107–128.
Türp, Jens: Zahnfegen, Zahnpinsel, Zahnputzhölzer. Zur Aktualität traditioneller Formen der
    Mund- und Zahnhygiene. In: Curare. Zeitschrift für Ethnomedizin und transkulturelle
    Psychiatrie 13 (1990), pp. 75–87.
Vigarello, Georges: Concepts of cleanliness. Changing attitudes in France since the Middle
    Ages. Cambridge; New York 1988.
Wilke, Jürgen: Grundzüge der Medien- und Kommunikationsgeschichte. 2nd ed. Köln; Wei-
    mar; Wien 2008.

The politics of intoxication. Dutch junkie unions fight against the ideal of a drug-free society, 1975–1990

Gemma Blok

Introduction

In 1982, in the Dutch city of Rotterdam, a local 'junkie union' organized a guerilla methadone programme. The junkies wanted to offer an emergency provision of this synthetic opiate to the large number of destitute heroin users in the streets, who often suffered acute withdrawal symptoms when they did not have the means to buy heroin. With the help of a sympathetic doctor and pharmacist, the junkie union was able to get three hundred pills of methadone each week. Two union members constantly carried an emergency stock, which they handed out to drug users whom they encountered in the streets, in buses or in trams, at any time, day or night. Ever since its foundation in 1980, the Rotterdam Junkie Union had argued for an unconditional supply of methadone. According to the union, the methodology in addiction treatment was 'outrageous' because of its one-sided insistence on abstinence.

Historically, in Dutch addiction treatment, the ties between professional carers and self-help groups of addicted clients had always been quite close. Before the Second World War, self-help organizations for alcoholics, such as the International Order of Good Templars, were actively involved in the institutional care for alcoholics. After 1945, Dutch institutions for addiction treatment worked closely together with the Alcoholics Anonymous. During the 1970s and 1980s, however, the relationship between the providers of addiction treatment and its new group of drug-using clients was rather strained.

At the time, organizations for drug users sprang up in various cities in the Netherlands. In the mid-1980s, there were some 15 to 20 groups, although some of them were quite small and were still at a formative stage.[1] They joined forces under the umbrella organization known as the Federation of Junkie Unions.[2] The biggest and most active organizations were, not surprisingly, based in Amsterdam and Rotterdam. These were the largest cities in the Netherlands with the largest number of drug users. The use of heroin was also quite visible in both cities.

During the 1970s and 1980s, an 'open drug scene' existed in Amsterdam and Rotterdam, where certain streets in the city centres were almost completely taken over by dealers and users. These streets were regarded as 'no-go

---

1   International Institute for Social History Amsterdam (henceforth IISG), MDHG archive, inv. no. 17. The folder 'Amsterdamse Junkiebonden' contains a leaflet listing all known junkie unions in existence between 1981–1987.
2   In Dutch: Federatie van Junkie Bonden (FJB).

areas' by many Dutch citizens.[3] In 1977, the 'Medical and Social Service for Heroin Users' (Medisch-sociale Dienst voor Heroïne Gebruikers, MDHG) was founded in Amsterdam, followed by the Junkie Union (Junkiebond) in Rotterdam in 1980. Both these interest groups for drug users are still very active today.

Compared to many other European countries, the Netherlands seem rather unique in that they had an active drug-user movement quite early on. Apart from Sweden, where a movement of drug users was already present during the latter half of the 1960s[4], there were few interest groups for drug users in other European countries before the 1990s. In Germany, the Dutch example inspired the institution of the first 'Junkiebund' in Kassel in 1982. Several others soon followed. However, this turned out to be a short-lived phenomenon; the 'Bünde' failed to attract a substantial constituency and withered away within a couple of years.[5]

British drug users did not really become visible until the mid 1990s, when they formed their own groups, were represented in various statutory organizations involved in the delivery of treatment services, and published magazines such as *The Users' Voice*.[6] In France as well, groups of drug users entered the stage at around 1990, in the wake of the HIV-Aids epidemic. Concern about this new public health problem greatly stimulated the formation of interest groups for drug users, who were especially vulnerable to infection with the HIV virus when they shared syringes to inject heroin.

This article will examine the views and actions of the Dutch junkie unions during the peak of heroin use in the Netherlands, roughly between 1975 and 1990. First of all, the origins and context of the early movement for clients in addiction treatment facilities will be sketched. What kind of therapies were the clients of addiction treatment exposed to during the 1970s, and how did the various drug user organizations come into existence? What caused the estrangement between carers and client organizations in addiction treatment?

To answer these questions, the main objectives and activities of the leading drug-user groups will be analysed. What exactly did they want to change and what kind of alternative health practices did they themselves experiment with? Finally, an attempt will be made to assess the influence of drug-user groups. Did they succeed in their efforts to transmit their views on the nature of intensive drug use and the best way to handle addicts based on their subjective expert experiences to policy-makers and professionals working in addiction treatment?

---

3   The Zeedijk in Amsterdam and the Kruiskade in Rotterdam.
4   Laanemets (2006).
5   Schmid (2003), p. 188.
6   Mold (2008), pp. 136 and 147.

Birth of the Dutch junkie unions during the 1970s

The Dutch approach to hard-drug users during the 1970s and early 1980s, when the drug-user groups were founded, was characterized by a strong ambivalence. The notion that the addict was a patient, not a criminal, had become the foundation of national and local policy by the mid 1970s. However, if we look at the actual treatment the addicts received, many of them were left uncared for. The existing institutions for addiction treatment were quite small and still trying to adjust to the explosion of drug use that was taking place at the time. Besides, treatment in the field strongly focused on abstinence. The temperance tradition in Dutch addiction treatment still reverberated in mission statements calling for a 'fight against addiction'.

The primary reaction of those in the field of addiction treatment to the new group of patients, the opiate addicts, was two-fold. Methadone was introduced in Holland during the late 1960s for the small number of people who had started to inject opium. At first, these programmes were quite liberal and non-committal, but as the heroin epidemic started to spread after 1972, the methadone programmes were transformed into stricter reduction programmes. A small number of therapeutic communities for addicts was created in addition to these methadone programmes.[7]

The national government supported the abstinence approach in addiction treatment. According to a consultative government body on health care and drug abuse, in a report from 1976, the only treatment of addicts that made any sense was 'one that principally aims to free the addict from drugs. If one offers the addict shelter and food, this only stimulates him to continue his lifestyle.' This choice of words is significant; implicitly, addiction was regarded not as a disease but as a lifestyle of choice.[8] The main Amsterdam institute for addiction treatment, the Jellinek, stated that addiction was 'an opportunity for personal growth'. The institute noted that it wanted to help only those who 'expressed a clear wish to be helped'.

Many addicts expressed no such wish and were not in contact with any form of addiction treatment. Instead, they lived in squats and shelters, or were forced to stay in prisons or psychiatric hospitals where they had to kick the habit. There is no legislation in the Netherlands that can force addicts to commit to institutional addiction treatment. The only way to have them committed against their will is through the Insanity Law, or through the legal system. Some prison directors were willing to provide addicted inmates with methadone, others were not. In Rotterdam there were about 3,000 to 3,500 drug users around 1980. An estimated 720 of them were taking part in a methadone programme, while 150 addicts were in a clinic or therapeutic community.[9] In Amsterdam, during the 1970s, only a couple of hundred clients a year took

---

7   About 10 therapeutic communities for drug addicts existed in Holland around 1980.
8   Blok (2008), p. 248.
9   Rotterdamse Junkiebond (1981).

part in one of the methadone programmes offered by the Jellinek. Taking into
consideration that the population of addicts amounted to about 8,000–9,000
people in Amsterdam around 1980, this number is not very high. Nationally,
the number of heroin addicts was estimated to be around 20,000 at the time.
Some 3,000–4,000 of them were on methadone.[10]

Care and shelter for homeless addicts was offered by private individuals
who often came from a countercultural background themselves. They created
drug consumption rooms, soup kitchens and day or night shelters. Their work
was commonly referred to as 'alternative addiction treatment'. Charitable religious organizations were quite active in creating this type of care for drug users as well. Many of these private and religious initiatives for addicts were financially supported by local town councils.

Looking for a 'third way'

The founding meeting of the MDHG took place on 2 May 1977 in the inner
city of Amsterdam. The setting was the home of concerned citizen and former
politician Johan Riemens. In the 1960s, Riemens had been the co-founder of
the Dutch Pacifist Socialist Party (PSP), a party that tried to escape from the
Cold War dichotomy between capitalism and communism. They campaigned,
amongst other ideals, for nuclear disarmament and advertised using a poster
that depicted a cheerful blond girl running naked through a meadow, sur-
rounded by cows. Now, sitting on a small platform, the ageing idealist Riemens spoke to the small group of people who had gathered in his house. They
had come there in response to an advertisement that Riemens had placed in a
national newspaper about the formation of a platform to help Amsterdam's
drug users.

At the meeting, Riemens talked about the misery of the heroin users he
observed around his house every day. He wondered whether professionals
working in addiction treatment had ever witnessed the degrading, tragic daily
lives of drug users. Did they even know what kind of life these people were
forced to live? Riemens accused the Dutch society in its approach to addiction
treatment of applying a philosophy of neglect. According to him, the implicit
assumptions ran something like this: Let's not affirm drug users in their lifestyle by helping them too readily. If they refuse to cooperate, then just let
them end up in the gutter. That will motivate them to quit the habit. The addict was thus caught between the police and prison on the one hand, and an
abstinence-oriented addiction treatment on the other. There should be a third
way here as well, Riemens argued: integrating hard-drug users back into society; supporting them whether they were using hard drugs or not; treating them

---

10 IISG, Federatie van Instellingen voor de Zorg voor Alcoholisten (FZA) archive, inv. no.
    210, 'Bezetting FZA gebouw door Junkiebonden'.

like 'normal' persons with specific problems, instead of stigmatizing and ex-
cluding them.[11]

Riemens' plea was received with great enthusiasm by the young and ambitious street-corner worker, August de Loor, who had been working in the
populous neighbourhoods of Amsterdam since the beginning of the 1970s. He
had closely witnessed the quick spread of heroin use amongst young people
with little education and few prospects. The atmosphere in those days, he remembers, was one of doom and disappointment. The flower power mood of
the 1960s had faded, and the younger brothers and sisters of the 'provos' (ac-
tivists) and hippies had to deal with rising unemployment and housing short-
ages.

In those days, a new group of people was discovering drugs, not sitting on
the grass in the Vondelpark, but hanging out in snack bars in the under-privileged parts of town. For a short while in 1972, heroin was handed out to potential new clients almost for free, as new dealers from South-East Asia tried to
enter the Dutch market. De Loor could see the results of the criminalization of
drugs around him every day. De Loor: 'These young people using drugs were
not the "lucky few"; they were the children of divorced parents, unemployed
fathers, the employees of illegal contractors and adolescents who had run
away from home. Their drug use was not financed by their parents. They had
to pay for it themselves, by legal or illegal means.'[12]

The fourteen individuals present at the founding meeting of the MDHG
in 1977 were a mixed group of people. Some of them were physicians and
volunteers working in 'alternative' addiction treatment facilities, such as night
shelters and walk-in centres. Others were members of interest groups for im-
migrants from Surinam. Some were actual drug users. In those early days, the
input from solicitors speaking on behalf of drug users was also quite important
at the MDHG.[13] The new organization worked from the home of Johan Riemens, who put the ground floor of his upmarket canal-side house at the dis-
posal of the MDHG. For several decades, the MDHG held its meetings, con-
sultations and walk-in hours at this house.

In Rotterdam, developments took exactly the opposite course: the initiative to form a junkie union was taken by drug users themselves, especially its
chairman Nico Adriaans (1957–1995), who then started to approach possible
supporters and sympathizers. One of his most successful alliances was with the
reverend Hans Visser, who was minister at St. Paul's Church in the centre of
Rotterdam, quite close to the central railway station. The station was struggling to deal with the influx of drug users and others on the fringes of society,
such as psychiatric patients, alcoholics and prostitutes. Adriaans simply approached Visser one day, asking if his church wanted to join forces with the
Junkie Union. Visser and Adriaans became close friends and together they

---

11   Riemens (1977).
12   Jonge (1997), p. 6.
13   Roosjen (2007), p. 7.

would initiate and coordinate many new activities for drug users. The Junkie Union also had its office at St. Paul's Church.

Visser described his friend, who died of AIDS in 1995, as a 'cultural rebel whose drug use was part of his resistance against the capitalist forces in society. Unfortunately, he was forced to discover that his resistance had resulted in a heroin addiction.'[14] According to him, Adriaans hated hypocrisy, bureaucracy, dishonesty and cheating.[15]

Both the Rotterdam Junkie Union and the MDHG were very active in securing support, making contact with national and local politicians, making good use of the media, and cooperating with universities. For example, in 1981, the Junkie Union was a guest of the Netherlands' most popular radio station for ten Fridays in a row, explaining its view on drug use and addiction treatment. Adriaans was in close contact with researchers working at the Institute for Preventive and Social Psychiatry at the Erasmus University in Rotterdam.

One of these researchers, Jean-Paul Grund, remembers how 'Nico saw his role as that of the tribesman who helped the scientist access and understand tribal culture. When I started working at the institute two years later, I was happy to be that scientist and Nico taught me a lot. For several years Nico worked on my study into the drug-taking rituals of heroin and cocaine users.'[16] Together with several other left-wing academics, Adriaans and Grund founded the 'United Front for the Renewal of Drug Policy'. In 1986, Adriaans left the Junkie Union to become a 'community field worker' at the Institute for Preventive and Social Psychiatry.

At the MDHG office in Amsterdam, students and academics from various universities were regularly welcomed as well to conduct research into the habits and lifestyles of drug users, and to transmit the expert knowledge about intensive drug users to researchers in the academic world. The drug-user groups also operated in close contact with each other. The MDHG and the Junkie Union held meetings together at Riemens' canal-side house, worked on publications together and coordinated their actions. All Dutch drug-user groups, moreover, were united under the banner of the above-mentioned Federation of Junkie Unions. Besides, both the MDHG and the Rotterdam Junkie Union also managed to gain financial support from their local city councils within a couple of years.[17] Meanwhile, smaller unions, such as those in Nijmegen and Groningen, were struggling to survive.

14   Visser (1996), p. 10.
15   Visser, 'Nico Adriaans 1957–1995', at http://www.aidsmemorial.nl (last access: Dec. 11th 2010).
16   Grund, 'Letter for Nico', at: http://www.ibogaine.desk.nl/adriaans.html (last access: Dec. 11th 2010).
17   Jonge (1997), p. 6; IISG, MDHG archive, inv. no. 17, folder 'Amsterdam Junkie Unions'.

Central themes and issues in the user groups

When looking at the writings and actions of various Dutch user groups of the
1970s, 1980s and early 1990s, it becomes obvious that their themes were quite
similar. The main goals, which will be elaborated below, can be summarized
as follows:

1. Acceptance of drug use and the drug user
2. Respectful treatment of drug users
3. More 'care' instead of 'cure' in addiction treatment

To start with the first goal: the dominant motive, the umbrella covering all activities, was the promotion of the 'acceptance model' (*aanvaardingsmodel*) of the
drug user, as it was called back then. The term, which came into vogue at
around 1980, is comparable to the German concept of 'akzeptierende Drogen-
arbeit', introduced there a decade later, at around 1990.[18] Today, we would
probably speak of 'harm reduction' to describe similar views on the treatment
of intensive drug users.

   According to the drug-user groups and their sympathizers, modern society
was to accept the fact that there would always be people who enjoyed drugs
and who wanted to use them, just as it had come to accept the fact that people
drank alcohol. A drug-free society was considered to be a utopian ideal and
the 'War on Drugs' the cause of many problems for heroin users.

   The junkie unions constantly fulminated against the police, especially after 1984, when more and more attempts were made to sweep the inner cities
of Amsterdam and Rotterdam clean. Drug users told stories about being
thrown into police vans and transported to plains outside of town.[19] The addicts also complained about being physically searched by the police in a rude
and aggressive manner. The dope that was found in their possession was often
thrown into a canal or otherwise destroyed. Comparisons with the Middle
Ages were often made in the drug user groups' pamphlets. 'Back in the old
days,' they wrote, 'whores, beggars, lepers and vagrants had to stay outside the
city gates. Today, junkies are the outcasts of society.'[20]

   Finally, according to the junkie unions and the MDHG, the Dutch government and the citizens of the Netherlands had to accept the fact that not all
intensive drug users were willing, or able, to stop using drugs. As Nico Adriaans put it in 1982:

> A junkie is not as deviant as many people think. There are many similarities between a
> junkie and a housewife addicted to Valium. But she does not need to go out and 'score'
> her dope, because her addiction is tolerated and even supported by her environment.
> Therefore, she does not become a 'junkie', while the user of illegal drugs does. A junkie

18 Schmid (2003), p. 204.
19 Visser (1996), p. 13.
20 MDHG/Junkiebond (1984), p. 2.

is not destroyed by heroin, but by everything else that comes along with the use of hero-in.[21]

An anonymous user stated in 1978: 'Nobody is willing to accept the fact that if a "junkie" were able to obtain his daily portion of dope in a normal fashion, he or she would be able to work and function just like anybody else. Many users would like that very much.'[22]

There were heated debates on the issue of accepting or countering opiate use. For instance, the Rotterdam Junkie Union organized a series of talks with psychiatrist Martien Kooyman, a well-known proponent of therapeutic communities for heroin addicts. They wanted to know, amongst other things, his views on Valium addiction in the Netherlands. Why were Valium addicts so easily supported in their habit by their doctors while heroin addicts could not be supplied methadone from their local General Practitioners (GPs)? Kooyman replied that he thought the phenomenon of Valium addiction was quite harmful as well. So why add another problem to it?

It seems that for many people at around 1980, it was still too early to accept the fact that heroin was there to stay. For instance, in a current affairs programme on Dutch television 'Here and now' (*Hier en nu*), reverend Hans Visser, the Protestant minister from Rotterdam and strong supporter of the local junkie union, discussed the Dutch drug policy with the Rotterdam head of police, J.A. Blaauw.[23] Visser argued that heroin use should be accepted as a given.

'It just happens,' he said. 'There are people who have their reasons for using it, just as there are people who use alcohol or Valium. They often suffer from hidden problems in their personal biography. Why should alcohol use be legal, and heroin use illegal?' Blaauw objected that alcohol abuse was a big problem in Dutch society as well. He asked: 'Just because we already have one big problem, do we have to accept the fact that we have another one as well, a heroin problem? Are we to surrender to this without resistance? That would be an admission of weakness.'

Visser reacted by stating that a dignified existence for all people should be the goal of all action. Heroin users deserved this as well, even if they continued to use drugs. We should accept the drug user and his deviant lifestyle, Visser argued, and support him so as to prevent social and physical degradation. Blaauw countered that according to him, it was not very dignified to simply give up on people. 'We do *not* give up on them!', Visser replied with pent-up rage. 'We want to save them from a life in the gutter.'

Other Protestant ministers supported this acceptance model of drug use and the drug user as well, possibly because it linked into their long tradition of religious philanthropy. Evangelical Christians had been active in the Netherlands since the nineteenth century in what they referred to as 'active Christi-

21   Rotterdamse Junkiebond/MDHG (1982), p. 15.
22   Stichting Streetcornerwork Amsterdam (1978), p. 16.
23   Instituut Beeld en Geluid, Hilversum, *Hier en Nu*, Nov. 28th 1983.

anity': trying to offer relief to the poor and the homeless by opening shelters in under-privileged areas and paying house visits to destitute families. The 'soldiers' working for the Salvation Army (which has been active in the Netherlands since 1887), for instance, and relief workers from comparable Protestant organizations, had always protested against the social exclusion of deviant groups. During the nineteenth and early twentieth century, they had taken mercy upon former prisoners and alcoholics. Now, they turned to a new group of people who were at the bottom of society's pecking order: heroin addicts.

In Amsterdam, reverend Douwe Wouters and his colleague Jelle van Veen strongly sympathized with the drug users flooding the streets of the Dutch capital at the time. They both worked for the Regenboog Foundation, a Protestant organization based in the city centre offering shelter to various groups of people, such as prostitutes and the homeless. Van Veen stated in 1979 in the local newspaper *Het Parool*: 'In order to be a good fieldworker, one should be able to shift one's boundaries and adjust to the addict's environment. This means, first of all, accepting his drug use. If a user does not want to kick the habit, then start by introducing some regularity into his life. A helper should not press an addict to stop using drugs.'[24]

In short, the root of the communication problem between 'official' addiction treatment and its clients, according to the 'junkies', was the result of Western society's drive for Utopia. Society, so they said, was trying to realize two impossible goals – the first to create a drug-free society. The second to save addicts from their disease.

Humour and respect

One of the aspects the junkie unions and the MDHG disliked most about addiction treatment was the way in which they were approached by those working in this field. In general, the members of the drug-user groups experienced the attitude of the professionals in addiction treatment as humiliating, arrogant, and full of pedantry.[25] The atmosphere, they reported, was one of distrust and seriousness; there were many complaints about the care-givers' lack of humour.[26]

One of the continuing complaints was a lack of knowledge about and understanding of the lifestyle and experiences of the drug user. Professionals, addicts claimed, behaved as 'office workers' with no feeling or sympathy for their clients. The official addiction treatment centres, such as the Jellinek, were experienced by many as strongholds of medical power and quite remote from their own lives.

24 *Het Parool*, August 3ʳᵈ 1979, 'Hulpverlener moet afkicken niet opdringen'.
25 Rotterdamse Junkiebond/MDHG (1982), p. 4.
26 Jezek (2000), p. 17.

Some psychiatrists working at the Jellinek or other institutions for addiction treatment were themselves quite young in the 1970s. Several *did* make an effort to enter into contact with the growing drug scenes in their cities at the end of the 1960s, for instance, by offering them practical advice on the long-term physical effects or combinations of drugs. A couple of psychiatrists working in addiction treatment in Amsterdam were even quite active in the Dutch campaign to decriminalize cannabis products.[27]

Still, although the gap between professionals and clients was not always as wide as the drug-user groups claimed, in many cases there probably were differences in age, gender and cultural background between the clients of addiction treatment and the professionals working in the field. In the 1970s, many social workers were (older) middle-class women, while many of the clients were (younger) men from a counter-cultural or lower-class background. One drug user remembered how he had to educate his social worker on drug abuse; she knew only alcohol and alcoholics. Together, they read the same book on drugs and addiction. Others were confronted by doctors who asked them whether they injected their cannabis, or who believed that LSD was as addictive as opium.[28]

A huge blemish for the junkie unions was the introduction of the term 'junkie syndrome', used to describe a pattern of behaviour ascribed to the chronic heroin addict. He would lie, cheat, steal and manipulate in order to get his hands on some dope. He was 'unbelievably cheeky and immodest', one psychiatrist wrote, 'and could never be trusted'.[29] In choosing the name 'Junkie Unions', heroin users re-appropriated the stigmatizing term 'junkie' and used it in a defiant manner.

The wish to keep a safe distance from the heroin-using client is certainly quite tangible in the manuals and articles of psychiatrists writing on addiction at around 1980. Much was written about the need for the therapist to stay in control in the therapeutic relationship. He was never to allow himself to be manipulated by the addict. Possibly, professionals working in addiction treatment were feeling a bit overwhelmed at the time because of the growing number of clients requesting help, or methadone.

Meanwhile, many drug users felt unjustly feared and distrusted. They did not deny the reality of this 'junkie behaviour', which indeed was quite common, as they admitted. However, this type of behaviour was caused not by the use of heroin itself, or by the inferior character of the addict, but mostly by the degrading life a heroin user was forced to live in a country where his drug of choice was forbidden, and thus quite expensive and hard to come by.

The junkie unions laid the blame for another type of unattractive behaviour of drug users at the door of addiction treatment. As professionals in the

27 This campaign was successful: the Opium Law of 1976 turned the possession of small amounts of hash and marihuana into an offense instead of a crime. Blok (2008), pp. 245–258.
28 Stichting Streetcornerwork Amsterdam (1978), pp. 8, 10.
29 Epen (1981), p. 56.

field had noticed as well, many 'junkies' would adopt the role of victim as they presented themselves to therapists or social workers. They told them tearful stories about their troubled lives and awful parents, and assured them that they really desperately wished to escape their horrible addicted existence.

The junkie unions noticed this kind of behaviour amongst their fellow drug users as well, with much dislike. Instead of regarding it as 'typical addict behaviour', they considered it to be a reaction to the therapeutic climate in addiction treatment. These clients were simply being strategic: they told their therapists exactly what they thought they wanted to hear. Didn't professionals in therapeutic communities always want to hear about hidden emotions and troubles in the family? Did they not stimulate their clients in 'scream therapy' sessions to get in touch with their suppressed anger towards their dominant fathers or cold mothers?

According to the MDHG, some users actually suffered from a 'detox syndrome'. For years they wandered from one therapeutic community or crisis centre to another. In this way, they learned exactly what to say – and what not to say – during an intake, how to behave during therapy sessions, and so on.[30] One thing they learned was not ever to admit that they were not completely convinced, deep down, that they wanted to stop using drugs for good. They knew that if they said that, all help would soon be withdrawn from them. According to the MDHG, this was the one big taboo in therapy-land. This created much deception on the part of the addict, who was constantly required to 'prove' his motivation to be helped.

Fighting for a 'low-threshold' methadone supply

The wish for more accessible and large-scale methadone maintenance was the central uniting issue for all drug-user groups. Junkies wanted care instead of cure. The 'treatment industry' was considered by them to be too one-sided in its focus on the promotion of abstinence. This resulted in a situation where the majority of addicts was forced to remain in the cold.

Many heroin users were critical of existing forms of addiction treatment. Methadone programmes often involved many rules such as urine testing, a prohibition of the use of other drugs, limited opening hours, and an obligation to partake in a reduction programme or psychotherapy. Therapeutic communities for addicts, in particular, were extremely unpopular. Clients felt humiliated and degraded by the hierarchical system in these institutions. On arrival, they were washed in a wooden laundry bowl, completely naked. This ritual was meant to clean them from their former junkie existence. Additionally, clients had to cut their hair, hand in their clothes and jewellery, wear an overall, and clean the kitchen and toilets. Any contact with friends or family members was not allowed for weeks or even months.

---

30 Stichting Streetcornerwork Amsterdam (1978), p. 24.

Meanwhile, they had to endure a continuing stream of critical and confrontational remarks on their behaviour by therapists and fellow-patients. These remarks were meant to break down their 'junkie identities'. In the opinion of the therapists, clients were often hiding behind a stereotypical 'character armour': the pathetic victim, or the tough street boy. The aim was to free the vulnerable person concealed within by shattering the addict's resistance to change and stimulate him to show his hidden emotions. Some clients reacted positively to this approach: they managed to run through the whole therapeutic programme and graduate after one or two years. Some graduates even became co-counsellors in a therapeutic community.

Quite often, on the other hand, the result of the intense regime was that people became agitated, depressed, scared or annoyed. Many clients ran away after one or two weeks. According to the junkie unions, there were many 'freaked-out' runaways, who felt desperate and confused after their stay in a therapeutic community. Some, they claimed, were even suffering from suicidal tendencies.[31] One of these runaways remembers how, during his short stay in a therapeutic community, he felt as if he were being dragged through the mud for the duration of his time there. 'My pride was hurt too much'.[32] Another person recounts with horror how he had to go through a shaming ritual that was often used in these therapeutic communities. It consisted of wearing a wooden 'sandwich board' around his neck for a couple of days, with the following text written on it: 'I am a creep because I am too scared to look into other people's eyes.'

Quite a few heroin users experienced these communities as a form of brainwashing, as legalized terror, or as a religious cult, where 'dope' was the enemy and where hysterical shouting and swearing at the drug-using 'sinners' served to exorcise this Devil.[33] Not all communities were as bad, however, according to the addicts. Whereas in some communities even a simple aspirin for a headache was completely taboo, in others a slow methadone reduction programme was possible. However, all communities had in common what addicts considered to be a very elitist regime. It favoured extrovert and eloquent clients, while many drug users were introverts or even slightly sociophobic.

'Alternative' forms of addiction treatment

The junkie unions worked hard to formulate and experiment with alternatives to this psychotherapeutic climate in addiction treatment. A soup kitchen for drug users was established in St. Paul's Church in Rotterdam, as well as day and night shelters.[34] In Amsterdam, the MDHG organized open consultation

---

31 Rotterdamse Junkiebond/MDHG (1982), p. 5.
32 Stichting Streetcornerwork Amsterdam (1978), p. 25.
33 Stichting Streetcornerwork Amsterdam (1978), p. 26; Rotterdamse Junkiebond/MDHG (1982), p. 5.
34 Visser (1996), p. 10.

hours a couple of nights a week, where drug users could get non-committal practical advice and support.

Christians and alternative addiction treatment workers further led initiatives such as walk-in shelters and drug consumption rooms, where addicts could buy drugs from house dealers, buy clean needles, get a medical check-up by a licensed doctor, and find a cheap and healthy meal and a warm bed. The MDHG had mixed feelings, however, as to these alternative initiatives. Although these places did serve as useful and necessary relief opportunities for many addicts who were out on the streets, they quite often turned into 'ghettos' and 'training institutes for junkies', according to the MDHG[35], which aimed at total liberation of the drug user from both the justice system, addiction treatment, *and* the drug scene. Ideally, in its view, a socially-adjusted drug user would be able to consume his methadone at home and live a normal life, independent of drug dealers, therapists and anti-social fellow users.

One of the first actions taken by the MDHG was to invite a group of local GPs to its office. These doctors came to be known as 'Doctor Ten'. Together, they supplied hundreds of heroin users with methadone. One of the Amsterdam 'methadone doctors', a psychiatrist called Hardenberg, described his views on addiction in an elaborate letter to his fellow doctors and psychiatrists in town on the occasion of his retirement from office in 1988.[36] At the end of the 1970s, Hardenberg had started prescribing methadone to some of his patients, because he had become 'convinced that heroin addiction truly was a disease that can afflict people of all kinds of character and from any social background'.

Methadone, according to Hardenberg, was a 'primary necessity of life' for addicts. This medicine enabled them to restore their confidence and gradually learn to control their addiction. Hardenberg considered it unjust that this category of patients was often treated by professionals with 'disgust, distrust and prejudice'. He argued that patients reacted to this hostile attitude with antisocial and egocentric behaviour. He concluded by saying that as a doctor, he had always tried to offer his addicted patients a stopping place in their chaotic lives instead of trying to 'discipline them with rules and regulations, like a police officer". He had wanted to offer them help and care 'without making judgements'.

Initiatives such as those described above were strongly discouraged at the time by institutions for addiction treatment, by the Royal College of Pharmacists, and by governmental health inspectors. They feared double prescriptions and overdosage. According to the junkie unions, however, what was known as the 'treatment industry' wanted to safeguard its monopoly on addiction treatment. An anti-institutional and anti-medical mentality was strongly present in the new social movements of drug users.

---

35   Stichting Streetcornerwork Amsterdam (1978), p. 38.
36   IISG, MDHG archive, inv. no. 11, Letter by L. Hardenberg, October 3rd 1988.

The idea of the MDHG was that 'Doctor Ten' would act as a lobby group to convince their fellow GPs that they should also start prescribing methadone to addicts. When this plan was unsuccessful, the MDHG managed to convince two doctors working for the Municipal Health Service to take up this task. These two doctors visited many local GPs to plead for more understanding for the plight in which addicts found themselves. Thousands of Amsterdam's heroin users were thus placed in general practices over the next couple of years.[37] In 1982, Stivema was founded. This organization was responsible for the registration of methadone clients and the prevention of double prescriptions. All parties involved in prescribing methadone took part in Stivema, such as the Jellinek, the Municipal Health Service, and various institutions for alternative addiction treatment. The MDHG was a member as well.

The MDHG then took on pharmacists, since they had to be willing to actually carry out the doctors' prescriptions. A group of lovely-looking ladies was selected from volunteers and social-workers-in-training, to hand out leaflets in Amsterdam's pharmacies about the nature, use and benefits of methadone. According to the leaflet, methadone enabled addicts to participate in society again as well as reducing aggression and criminality. The MDHG was hoping that pharmacists would be more willing to listen to these ladies than to 'a rough fellow in a squatter's outfit'.[38]

In Amsterdam, the relationship between the local city government, the Municipal Health Service and the MDHG seems to have been quite fruitful in the beginning, at least until the middle of the 1980s. The alderman for health affairs, Wim Polak, even invited August de Loor, as a representative of the MDHG, to advise him on the introduction of 'community methadone centres' in various neighbourhoods in Amsterdam. These centres were established by the Municipal Health Service from 1982 onwards in order to offer heroin users the opportunity to collect their methadone close to their homes, and receive advice, guidance, social and medical support at the same time. In some areas, these new centres met with stiff resistance from the inhabitants, who did not like the idea of 'junkies' in their neighbourhood. De Loor was able to bring some calm to this heated atmosphere, providing realistic information to these worried citizens, and thus became a valued advisor to the city council.[39]

In Rotterdam, the Junkie Union and the city council had a more rocky relationship. In 1981, the union met with the (socialist) mayor, André van der Louw, and an alderman of the city. At first, this meeting seemed to have positive results. The mayor himself paid a visit to a shelter for young prostitutes, along with the director of the Rotterdam Municipal Health Service. Soon after, an accessible methadone maintenance programme was set up at this shelter, but it was not nearly enough to service all heroin users in the city. Renewed efforts to expand the low-threshold methadone programmes were less

37 Jonge (1997), p. 10.
38 Jonge (1997), p. 8.
39 Jonge (1997), p. 9.

successful. The Junkie Union then occupied the office of the Rotterdam city council's advisor on drug affairs. This was the start of a long and troubled relationship between the city and the Junkie Union.[40]

In Nijmegen, much to the annoyance of the local junkies, the only methadone programme around was run by the psychiatric wing of a local general hospital. It consisted of a short-term reduction programme. The client would get his methadone for a period of twelve days only, in decreasing amounts. He had to go to the clinic every day to take his methadone pills under supervision. This programme, according to the local junkie union, was only effective for a very small group of drug addicts. Others lied and cheated, faking motivation to stop using drugs in order to get into the programme – to at least get their hands on some methadone in times of need. Many clients travelled to Amsterdam to score methadone on the black market.

Local doctors in smaller Dutch towns were often afraid to prescribe methadone because they were unfamiliar with addiction treatment or because they feared an increase of addicts and possible accompanying aggressive behaviour. This fear was not unjustified. In Arnhem, for instance, a venturesome doctor and pharmacist had actually had bad experiences in prescribing methadone. They started to experiment with this at the end of the 1960s, in order to help the small group of opium addicts in the area. However, when the number of heroin users started to increase, they suddenly had to deal with a problem on a different scale, as well as with impatient and aggressive clients. Besides, the large number of drug users in the doctor's waiting room and in the pharmacy began to scare away other customers.[41]

Still, in the course of the 1980s, methadone prescription steadily became more common. The Dutch government changed its views as well. Sometimes, it was now argued by policy-makers and health inspectors, another approach made sense in addiction treatment, besides that of freeing the addict from his drug abuse. Prevention of social degradation, it was argued, could also be a legitimate goal of treatment. By the early 1990s, methadone had become a cornerstone of Dutch addiction treatment. In part, this has been the result of the lobbying by the drug-user groups of the 1970s and 1980s. Junkies closely cooperated with the local Municipal Health Services, with sympathetic general practitioners, and with volunteers and professionals who were experimenting with an alternative kind of addiction treatment. Together, they made a strong plea for an acceptance model in drug-addiction treatment, with low-threshold methadone maintenance. Certainly, this had an impact on local and national policy. But the move towards harm reduction methods was the result of other considerations as well, such as the need to reduce drug-related crime and inconvenience for Dutch citizens and curb the growing unrest in cities such as Amsterdam and Rotterdam.[42]

40   Visser (1996); Bos/Jong/Kleer (1983), pp. 8–11.
41   Blok (2007), pp. 175 and 176.
42   As is argued in Blok (2008).

Conclusion

After 1977, Dutch interest groups for drug users thus dedicated themselves to transmitting practical, emotional and subjective knowledge about drug abuse and addiction which, in many ways, questioned the existing specialist knowledge in addiction treatment. The new socially-minded Dutch movement for drug users was very active during the 1980s. This was the result of the dedication shown by many persons involved, both the drug users themselves and those who sympathized with them. However, the support which the junkie unions encountered in the Netherlands was probably crucial as well. Many citizens, journalists, individual doctors and politicians lent an ear to the call of the junkies, in contrast to Germany where the 'Junkiebunden' withered away quite soon. The German junkies had presented themselves at several conferences held by institutes for drug research and addiction treatment, but their appearance only evoked irritation.[43]

In the Netherlands, the results of the many meetings and contacts with institutions, professionals and politicians certainly were not always satisfactory, in the opinion of the drug-user groups. Still, they did find a sufficiently large audience to keep going and feel at least a little encouraged. At least here, the junkies were invited to offer their opinions and attend meetings. In the large cities, they were supported financially. They encountered many like-minded people amongst left-wing academics and 'alternative' relief workers in addiction treatment. Besides, the user groups were willing to cooperate with each other as well. Thus, they proved to be very active and successful in gathering support and making their voices heard.

The junkie unions and the MDHG presented themselves as trade unions. Looking back on their views and actions now, this label seems rather limited. During those pioneering days, the user groups can truly be considered as 'new social movements'. They argued for a broad social change: the Opium Law was to be abolished and the stigmatization and social exclusion of drug users had to end.[44] Their views, issues and constituency were largely rooted in the counter-cultural movement of the 1960s, and they concerned themselves with the common themes of many other new social movements of the day: advancing individual freedom and well-being. In this sense, they can be compared to the women's movement, the movement for more humane psychiatric treatment and the gay liberation movement.

One very important goal of the junkie unions and the MDHG has been reached: methadone maintenance has become very accessible. Even before the AIDS epidemic created a panic, the number of methadone programmes and doctors willing to prescribe methadone had started to rise. By 1990, almost half of all hard-drug users was on methadone and the new philosophy of 'harm reduction' was becoming quite popular. According to this philosophy,

---

43   Schmid (2003), p. 188.
44   Rotterdamse Junkiebond/MDHG (1982), p. 2.

the aim of treatment is not to put an end to drug use, but to ameliorate the adverse social, medical and psychological effects of drug use. Today, about 12,500 people are enrolled in a methadone programme. This is almost half of all known problematic hard-drug users in the Netherlands, the number of which seems to have stabilized at about 25,000 people. Many methadone clients combine their use of methadone with regular or occasional use of cocaine, base-cocaine, heroin, alcohol or benzodiazepines. About 600 people partake in a heroin maintenance project.

In retrospect, the main cause for the estrangement between clients and healers in addiction treatment in the 1970s and 1980s, was the fact that both parties did not agree on the aim of addiction treatment. Most professional healers were working from the paradigm of abstentionism, while many clients felt they needed help and support even if they continued their drug use. The drug user groups at the time were fighting for an acceptance model of the drug user, a forerunner of the modern harm reduction paradigm. In this way, the junkie unions and the MDHG differed from traditional client organizations like the International Order of Good Templars, the Alcoholics Anonymous and Narcotics Anonymous. These organizations were strongly in favour of abstentionism as well.

Today in 2010, the heroin epidemic in Holland has passed its peak. The number of young new users is quite small and those who started their careers as addicts in the 1970s and 1980s are in their fifties or even sixties now. Many have died from an overdose, AIDS, or other health problems. With the average age of the Dutch hard-drug user rising, the number of deaths is on the increase as well. The coordinator of the National Support Group for Drug Users[45] – a national organization which has existed since the early 1990s – is now in training to arrange funerals.[46] In several places, hostels exist especially for elderly drug users, who are allowed to use their rooms. Heroin is provided for them by the hostel personnel. The occupants are allowed to go out, score some cocaine, and use this at home.

Care is now officially just as important in Dutch addiction treatment as cure. The chronic nature of addiction has become accepted and 'formulating a strong wish to be helped' is no longer a basic criterion in the selection of clients. Addicts who avoid care are considered to be a legitimate group of clients as well. The new socially-minded movement for drug users did not succeed, however, in putting a stop to the War on Drugs, or end the use of force against addicts by the police and the justice system. On the contrary, in the course of the 1990s, the possibilities in the Netherlands for the forced treatment and imprisonment of troublesome addicts have grown.

Furthermore, a new and quite different type of client movement in addiction treatment today suggests that perhaps the most fundamental goal of the junkie unions was never reached: the acceptance of drug users as free persons

---

45 In Dutch: the 'Landelijk Steunpunt Druggebruikers' (LSD).
46 Gerritsen (2009), p. 10.

with their own agency. Interestingly, nowadays in the Netherlands, a growing criticism from drug users is that methadone maintenance excessively dominates addiction treatment. Users complain that they are brushed aside when they indicate that they want to give it a try and stop taking drugs altogether. One former hard-drug user, Keith Bakker, has even filed a complaint against the Jellinek for refusing to help him properly. The only treatment they offered was methadone maintenance, he claims, when he came asking for their help in trying to stop using drugs. He went to an English rehabilitation clinic and did manage to stop his drug abuse, after almost twenty years of living on the streets, using heroin, alcohol and cocaine. He now runs his own private institute for addiction treatment, which is very successful in the Netherlands.[47]

The final aim of the junkies, in retrospect, was to create a completely different approach to addiction treatment, where the client is in charge and professionals adopt a helpful and empathetic attitude. Basically, the message the junkie unions and the MDHG were sending to addiction treatment facilities was that they should accept intensive drug users for who they *really* were, in their own view: drug users who had once had their reasons for starting to experiment with intoxication; who were now entertaining an intense love-hate relationship with their drug of choice, over which they have lost control; but who would get out of this dysfunctional relationship on their own terms only and in their own time. Pressure to change was futile and did not help in shaping a constructive therapeutic relationship. However, help should be on offer when the addict himself felt ready to change. But only the drug user could save himself – or not. Of course, this was asking a lot from a field which was created to convert addicts into new abstainers and was by its nature geared towards interventionism like all health care.

Many who were active in drug-user groups, however, did not regard drug abuse as an illness. According to them, drug abuse was not simply a terrible affliction one desperately wanted to get rid of. The situation was much more complex. Intensive drug use was a habit with which users often had a love-hate relationship.[48] On the one hand they desperately wanted to stop using drugs; on the other, they didn't. In spite of this tiresome predicament, many intensive drug users did not want to be regarded either as patients or as poor wretches. Today, however, addiction is seen in the Netherlands and elsewhere as a genetically and neurologically-based disease, tending towards chronicity. The user groups did not succeed in changing this medical paradigm of addiction.

They did succeed, however, in convincing people that junkies can be accepted as equal interlocutors deserving a say in the shaping of health knowledge and health practices in addiction treatment. The junkie unions were able

47   Bakker/Verdonschot (2008).
48   IISG Amsterdam, MDHG archive, inv. no. 12, 'Zo ken ik er nog wel een paar', memorandum on forced treatment, 1984.

to show, by their actions and writing, that hard-drug users could do much more than cheat, lie, steal and manipulate.

Grund, a close friend and colleague of Nico Adriaans, remembers meetings they had with representatives of all political parties in the Dutch parliament and with high-ranking officials within the Ministry of Health.

> They were flabbergasted … They had never engaged in a serious conversation with a drug user before [...] Now, here, they were confronted with an eloquent speaker, who debunked dangerous 'junkie syndrome' mythology, taught them the basics of street life and demanded sensible, pragmatic policies and services, such as 'low threshold' methadone maintenance. [...] Yet, he was … ahum ah … well … a junkie.[49]

In all probability, the junkie unions represented the 'elite' of the addict population. They were often better educated or more eloquent and probably less troubled by other psychiatric problems compared to some of their fellow users. Still, for this reason, they were able to improve the image of the heroin user and contribute to one of their main goals: the destigmatization of the drug user.

Bibliography

Bakker, Keith; Verdonschot, Leon: Pushing the limits. Het leven van Keith Bakker. Amsterdam 2008.

Blok, Gemma: Van 'zedelijke verheffing' tot 'harm reduction'. Verslavingszorg in Arnhem en Nijmegen, 1900–2000. In: Vijselaar, Joost et al (eds.): Van streek. 100 jaar geestelijke gezondheidszorg in Zuid-West Gelderland. Utrecht 2007, pp. 152–192.

Blok, Gemma: Pampering 'needle freaks' or caring for chronic addicts? Early debates on harm reduction in Amsterdam, 1972–1982. In: Social History of Alcohol and Drugs 22 (2008), no. 2, pp. 243–261.

Bos, Jannie; Jong, Wouter de; Kleer, Ricardo de: Nood breekt wet. Over methadonverstrekking door de Rotterdamse Junkiebond in de periode november 1981 tot 28 oktober 1982. Rotterdam 1983.

Epen, Hans van: Compendium drugsverslaving en alcoholisme: diagnostiek en behandeling. Amsterdam 1981.

Gerritsen, Martien: Uitvaart voor gebruikers. In: Mainline. Drugs, gezondheid en de straat (2009), no. 4, pp. 10–12.

Jezek, Rob: Recht op roes. Druggebruikers en belangenbehartiging. Alkmaar 2000.

Jonge, Louis de: Twintig jaar in een roes van overwinning. Belangenvereniging Druggebruikers MDHG 1977–1997. Amsterdam 1997.

Laanemets, Leili: Organisation among drug users in Sweden. Nordic Centre for Alcohol and Drugs. In: NAD Publications 49 (2006), pp. 105–130.

Medisch-sociale Dienst voor Heroïne Gebruikers (MDHG); Junkiebond: Zeedijk Dossier. Amsterdam 1984.

Mold, Alex: Heroin. The treatment of addiction in twentieth-century Britain. Dekalb, Ill. 2008.

Riemens, Johan: De heroïne epidemie: een aanklacht en een recept. Amsterdam 1977.

Roosjen, Geja: Dertig jaar scoren, drugscene, MDHG 1977–2007. Lelystad 2007.

---

49 Grund, 'Letter for Nico', at: http://www.ibogaine.desk.nl/adriaans.html (last access: Dec. 11th 2010).

Rotterdamse Junkiebond: Zwartboek Methadon. Rotterdam 1981.

Rotterdamse Junkiebond; Medisch-socialer Dienst voor Heroïne Gebruikers (MDHG): Verslag van tien gesprekken tussen Martien Kooyman en leden van de Junkiebonden. Rotterdam 1982.

Schmid, Martin: Drogenhilfe in Deutschland. Entstehung und Entwicklung 1970–2000. Frankfurt/Main 2003.

Stichting Streetcornerwork Amsterdam: Zes vooruit naar Hattem of terug naar de gevangenis. Amsterdam 1978.

Visser, Hans: Perron Nul. Opgang en ondergang. Zoetermeer 1996.

'Give them practical lessons': Catholic women religious and the transmission of nursing knowledge in late nineteenth-century England[1]

Carmen M. Mangion

> Be particular about the Nursing lectures. Make them learn by heart and also give them practical lessons, putting on leeches, going to bed to be poulticed, sheets changed, etc.[2]

Introduction

Nursing knowledge has sharply divided medical and nurse practitioners in the past and continues to challenge educators and historians in the present. In the latter half of the nineteenth-century, nurses, medical men and philanthropists in England bickered over what sorts of knowledge was necessary for nurses. These debates hinged on differences of opinion with regards to the profession-alisation of nursing, gendered ideals of womanhood and authority in hospital spaces. Central to these debates was the concept of vocation which implied that nursing was more than an occupation, but a calling. Many accepted that good moral character was the keystone of a good nurse and that training in obedience as well as nursing tasks was necessary. But the medicalisation of nurse training was a point of marked divisions. Those who sought a more pro-fessional nursing status fought for a medicalised and scientific nursing educa-tion and a registration process that would identify nurses who had passed through a rigorous process of examination. Others opposed professionalisa-tion on the grounds that nursing was a vocation and a medicalised education and registration would turn nursing into a 'mere' occupation. Medical practi-tioners faced another set of concerns as they feared that their own authority and power on the wards would be challenged by more formally-trained nurses. The emotive rhetoric of these debates persistently surfaced in the medical and the nascent nursing press, sometimes spilling over into the national press.[3]

---

1   I would like to express my gratefulness to the religious institutes and archivists that al-lowed me access to the private archives of their congregations: Little Company of Mary Congregational Archives; General Archives of the Union of the Sisters of Mercy of Great Britain; Central Congregational Archive of the Poor Servants of the Mother of God; Ar-chives of the Poor Servants of the Mother of God 'Instituto Mater Dei', Rome; Archives of the Daughters of Charity of St Vincent de Paul; Archives of the Filles de la Croix.
2   Little Company of Mary Congregational Archives (henceforth LCM), Book I, Undated letter from Mary Potter to M. Rose (Mary) Moules, p. 107.
3   Baly (1973); Dingwall/Rafferty/Webster (1988).

Within this heated context, nineteenth-century Catholic women's religious congregations began opening and operating hospitals, convalescent homes and infirmaries as well as engaging in domiciliary nursing in England. Their contributions to the medical marketplace rarely appears in the historiography of health care in part due to the dominance of the Nightingale versions of nursing history where formally trained nurses were heralded as pioneers of modern nursing practices but also because of the predominance of institutional histories which have focused on larger, more prominent hospitals and the marginalisation of the relationship between religion and medical care.[4] The research for this paper is part of a larger project that examines Catholic contributions to the medical marketplace in nineteenth-century Britain in particular highlighting the significance of religion, gender and locality to the development of Catholic health care services.

This essay shall focus on the 'practical lessons' women religious functioning as sister-nurses gave, received and utilised.[5] These 'practical lessons' were an integral component of their informal networks of nursing knowledge. First, in a brief overview, the patterns of home and institutional provision delivered by female Catholic religious congregations will be identified. Significantly, this will focus on how the perceived needs of the patients related to the development of health care practices and knowledge. Next, the focus of this paper will shift to examine the methods of transmission of medical knowledge. For much of the nineteenth century (and into the twentieth), women religious acquired and disseminated health care knowledge in a variety of ways. Some attended nurse training courses in the growing number of British nursing training schools but much of the acquisition of knowledge of health practice occurred via informal networks of knowledge whereby health care practices were transmitted from sister to sister or from doctor to sister. These networks of knowledge were local and international and included the nursing sisters, the doctors and the patients. This paper will focus on these informal networks, examining how nursing sisters obtained information about health practices.

Extant material from the archives of most religious congregations are for the most part silent on the education the sisters obtained for their work as nurses in the nineteenth century. It is difficult to ascertain whether formal curriculums or instructions existed or not; many documents have been lost or

4   The term 'trained nurse' in this essay will be used to denote nurses who obtained a hospital certificate which signified that they had received hospital training.
5   Catholic women interested in religious life in the nineteenth century had two options: contemplative or active religious life. The contemplative life was one of prayer lived in an enclosed community. Women who entered this mode of life were called nuns and took solemn vows and lived in communities called orders. The active religious life was also one of prayer but included activities that occurred outside convent walls such as teaching, nursing and visiting the sick. Most of the women who managed health care institutions were from this cohort. These women, called sisters, took simple vows and lived in communities called congregations. Women religious is a general term used to refer to both nuns and sisters. In this essay, the terms 'nursing sister' and 'sister-nurses' will be used to refer specifically to women religious who nursed.

destroyed in fits of spring cleaning and organisation. The majority of the evidence for this essay was found in the archives of three congregations, the Poor Servants of the Mother of God which ran Providence Free Hospital in St Helens, the Religious Sisters of Mercy which managed the Hospital of St John and St Elizabeth's in London and the Little Company of Mary whose sisters acted as domiciliary nurses in England. Through a close reading of the texts, mainly correspondence, house diaries and annual reports, we can develop a picture of how health care knowledge was obtained, transmitted and employed by nursing sisters. While this paucity of sources makes it all the more difficult to ascertain the degree of nursing knowledge obtained by the majority of sisters, it still gives a sense of the steps taken to educate sister-nurses. For these three congregations, nursing knowledge was important, not only in terms of patient care, but also as a means of competition with non-Catholic institutions. It is clear that some congregation leaders thought it important that their sister-nurses be acknowledged as 'trained nurses'.

Catholic health care

Almost all of the 108 Catholic women's religious institutes residing in nineteenth-century England provided some sort of basic health care provision, the most frequent form was visiting the sick poor. Twenty-seven provided significant medical services; seventeen were involved in institutional care while the remaining ten provided medical services for patients in their homes. In total, women religious managed or nursed in thirty-five primarily medical institutions as well as provided domiciliary nursing care. The institutions can be grouped into two categories: by general hospitals and specialist institutions. Only four were included in the general hospital category and were listed in "Burdett's Hospital Annual and Year Book of Philanthropy" in 1900. These included the 60-bed Providence Free Hospital which was located in the industrial town of St Helens, Lancashire. Over fifty per cent of the cases treated at Providence were related to factory injuries, fractures, burns and scalds, pneumonia, pleurisy, bronchitis and rheumatism. The Daughters of Charity of St Vincent de Paul (and later the Servants of the Sacred Heart of Jesus) nursed in the French Hospital and the Italian Hospital. The sisters did not manage these hospitals; they were hired nurses, which was contrary to the pattern of the other institutions women religious managed in England. The Italian Hospital was a seventy-bed hospital and the French hospital had fifty beds as well as a dispensary. The Servants of the Sacred Heart of Jesus made a foundation to Aberdare, Wales in 1881 where they managed and nursed in the purpose built hospital donated by the Marquis of Bute. The ground floor contained a dispensary, a men's ward with three beds, an operating room with an apparatus for bringing into use Lister's antiseptic treatment, a day room for convalescing patients and a room fitted with ophthalmoscope for examinations of the throat, ears and eyes. The upstairs included female and children's wards with four beds, a bathroom with Maughan's Patent Geysers and cold and hot water baths.[6] These institutions would have competed directly with other local voluntary hospitals.

The next thirty-one specialist institutions were less likely to have many competitors. They can be divided into three broad categories. The first category includes institutions for those who suffered from incurable diseases. For example, the "Catholic Directory" of 1900 noted that St Mary's and St Margaret's both run by Dominican sisters were for 'female patients of good character afflicted with incurable diseases'.[7] St John and St Elizabeth's hospital was a fifty-bed hospital in London managed by the Sisters of Mercy. The annual report of 1898 noted that

> For more than forty years the work has been carried on as a refuge for the dying and as a means of restoring to health and active life to those who otherwise would probably have either died or been permanently crippled.[8]

What this statement made clear was that St John and St Elizabeth's set out to avoid competing with Protestant institutions. The 1864 annual report noted that the hospital for incurables met a 'well-known want' without 'clashing or entering into rivalry with other hospitals'.[9]

The next set of institutions were a bit more eclectic. Their patients would be those with mental and physical ailments that made independent life in nineteenth-century England difficult. Patients in these institutions would have needed constant physical and medical care. But also this list includes ophthalmic hospitals and infirmaries for children which typically required more short-stay medical treatment. The remaining grouping includes institutions for convalescing patients. St Joseph's Convalescent Home opened its doors in 1888 and within a week, the sisters were nursing eight male and female patients. By 1900, it contained eighty beds and annually treated 613 patients.[10] Their focus seems to have been on 'diseases of the chest', which likely meant tuberculosis, a prolific killer in the nineteenth century.

It is significant that the majority of institutions managed by women religious were specialist institutions which treated the chronically ill, those who needed permanent or long-term care or those who were convalescing. As will be discussed in the final section of this essay, in many cases it was not interventionist medical procedures that these patients needed, but therapeutic care that relied on bed rest, dietetics or pain relief. In addition, given the charitable imperative of many religious congregations, many patients would have been

---

6   *Aberdare Times* (26 March 1881). I am thankful to Geoff Morgan and Denise Jones, local
      historians of Aberdare who brought this article to my attention.
7   The Catholic Directory (1900), p. 535.
8   London Metropolitan Archives (henceforth LMA), SC/PPS/093 26.1, Hospital of St John
      and St Elizabeth Annual Report (1898), pp. 8–10.
9   General Archives of the Union of the Sisters of Mercy of Great Britain, Handsworth,
      0/305/2/157, Hospital of St John of Jerusalem and St Elizabeth of Hungary Annual Report (1865), p. 5.
10   Burdett (1901), p. 630.

the working-class poor. An analysis of the patient register of St Joseph's Hospital in Preston indicates that of those patient's whose occupation was recorded, all but ten could be broadly defined as working class. The majority of patients were labourers, cotton weavers and domestic servants.[11] John Woodward has argued that British hospitals avoided admitting the chronically sick or incurable, leaving the state (through the poor law) to care for these patients.[12] Significantly, the medical institutions managed by women religious were viable alternatives to Poor Law hospitals. As this next section will show, the perceived needs of these patients were relevant to the acquisition of health care knowledge and the development of clinical practices by sister-nurses.

Informal networks of knowledge

For Catholic women religious, networks of knowledge were local and international, connecting religious congregations in England with local doctors and nurse training schools as well as religious congregations on the continent and in Ireland. These networks included the nursing sisters, the doctors and the patients. For the purposes of this chapter, informal methods includes practical training by the patient's bedside as well as medical lectures on the wards and in the classroom, by sisters and doctors, but this knowledge, though sometimes examined internally, did not necessarily lead to a nursing certificate. (Formal methods of nurse training, which will not be discussed in this chapter, led to a hospital certificate and denoted a 'trained nurse'.)

European networks

In the nineteenth century, medical knowledge was not disseminated in a uniform or a consistent fashion. Even within the same congregation, a mix of informal and formal methods of transmission occurred which reflected the multifarious 'networks' of nursing knowledge. Religious congregations cannot be easily divided into those that utilised informal training and those that accessed formal training. Most congregations used both, training some sister-nurses informally and others more formally. One such congregation was the Poor Servants of the Mother of God. This congregation, founded in London by Frances (Fanny) Taylor (1832–1900) in 1869 developed a wide range of charitable in-

---

11 Lancaster Record Office, St Joseph's Patient Register, 1879–1900. Of the 516 patients treated from 1879–1900, only 202 had an occupation listed. For a fuller discussion of Catholic medical institutions and their patients, see my forthcoming book "Medicalised Places, Sacred Spaces: Faith, Philanthropy and Catholic Health Care in Nineteenth-Century Britain".
12 Woodward (1974).

stitutions including Providence Free Hospital.[13] Taylor, in her youth, had been
a member of the second cohort of nurses who joined Florence Nightingale in
the Crimea.[14] Prior to her departure for the Crimean War in 1854, she had
taken a short nurse training course at St George's Hospital in London. That
personal experience of training and her exposure to nursing in the Crimea
likely convinced her that her religious sisters would benefit from similar nurse
training.

   Nurse training for the Poor Servants proceeded at a variety of levels. Two
sisters, Sister M. Clare (Margaret) Doyle (1852–1880) and M. Lucy (Maria)
Forrestal (1856–1944) were initially sent to the Augustinian convent at Louvain, to the Grand Hospital, for two months for nursing training in November
1876.[15] Evidence of their training programme is sparse but extant correspondence indicates it included comforting and feeding the sick poor as well as the
study of dispensary skills (the 'mixing of medicines') and surgical nursing. The
two sisters remained an additional few weeks training at the hospital at the
suggestion of the Superior of the Louvain convent to 'learn a little more surgery and at the same time keep themselves up to date with all sort of things
which would be very useful'.[16] The hospital in Louvain catered to the medical
needs of the sick poor, and thus the skills taught, making a patient comforta-
ble, the use of dietetics and the compounding of medicines would be useful in
visiting the poor. The surgical nursing skills would be utilised in a hospital setting.

   Utilising European convent networks for learning skills was not an unusual practice. Such convent networks were an important means of 'professional expertise, practical information and fellowship'.[17] The Bermondsey Sisters of Mercy who joined Florence Nightingale nursing in the Crimea were led
by Mother Mary Clare (Georgiana) Moore (1814–1874) whose medical experience was obtained nursing the poor in Dublin infirmaries and during cholera
epidemics. But the Bermondsey sisters were not experienced in military nursing, so, on their way to the Crimea, they stopped in Paris to visit the Daughters
of Charity of St Vincent de Paul at Rue de Bac and sought their advice on
nursing in the battlefields. The Daughters of Charity were experienced in military nursing: they were frequently portrayed on the battlefield and were likely
the cohort of 'Sisters of Charity' that war correspondent William Howard Rus-

---

13   They also managed orphanages, night schools and refuges for penitents along with the
     ubiquitous visiting the sick poor. By the end of the nineteenth century, the congregation
     operated twelve convents, seven in Britain, three in Ireland and two on the continent and
     included 199 professed sisters.
14   Devas (1927), p. 24.
15   Central Congregational Archive of the Poor Servants of the Mother of God (henceforth
     SMG), B/1, Annals of the Congregation of the Poor Servants of the Mother of God Mary
     Immaculate in England (c. 1865–1880), p. 26.
16   Archives of the Poor Servants of the Mother of God 'Istituto Mater Dei Convent', Rome,
     Letter from M. Clare Doyle to M. Magdalen Taylor dated 7 January 1877; Letter from
     Sister Rosalie to M. Magdalen Taylor dated 27 January 1877.
17   Mangion (2008), p. 173.

sell (1820–1907) praised in his article in *The Times* which highlighted the 'disgraceful' conditions in the British military hospitals. Though no details are extant of the knowledge that was exchanged, the Sisters of Mercy, on the recommendation of the Daughters of Charity, purchased surgical instruments to use in the Crimea perhaps indicating the nature of the training they received.[18]

Numerous continental congregations like the Daughters of Charity of St Vincent de Paul and the Augustinians in Louvain were well versed in hospital nursing. Colin Jones's research on the Daughters of Charity of St Vincent de Paul in seventeenth-century France has suggested that they were well-respected as hospital administrators and were regarded as 'independent medical practitioners in their own right'.[19] Their medical skills were much needed: they worked as sister-apothecaries growing their own medicinal herbs, performed minor operations (in doctor-less rural locales) and by the early eighteenth century, doctors and hospital administrators 'seemed to accept the important medical role which the sisters had assumed'.[20] The effectiveness of the nursing work of women religious on the continent was reinforced in the mid-nineteenth century when a report on the conditions of the military hospital at Scutari and a comparison to the nursing being done by the French Sisters of Charity led to the question published in *The Times*: 'Why have we no Sisters of Charity?'.[21]

The apprenticeship model

The training the Poor Servants received at the Augustinian Hospital in Louvain provided the necessary skills for their work visiting the sick poor. The visiting work done in St Patrick's in Soho was first of all religious: sisters went to the homes of local Catholics and confirmed that children were baptised and sent to Catholic schools and encouraged families to attend Mass and approach the Sacraments.[22] The Poor Servants were following the dictates of their spiritual vocation. They were instructed in their 'Rule and Constitutions', the binding documents of religious congregations, that

> Whilst striving to help all in their temporal miseries, and by consoling the afflicted, restraining the intemperate and reconciling those at variance, the Sisters are promoting peace, their greatest care shall, however, be for immortal souls, and they shall endeavour in all they do, to lead all gently to accept religious instruction, to approach the Sacraments, to abandon the occasions of sin, and to lead Christian lives.[23]

18   Green (1994/95), p. 123.
19   Jones: Imperative (1989), pp. 137, 156. See also Jones: Sisters (1989).
20   Jones: Imperative (1989), pp. 113, 192–197.
21   *The Times* (14 October 1854), p. 7, 'Hospital Assistants in the East'.
22   SMG, 'First Houses of the Congregation–Accounts of Foundation–Sisters' Reminiscences', p. 7.
23   SMG, Rule & Constitutions of the Poor Servants of the Mother of God and the Poor (1892), Chapter XIV.

Despite the focus on the spiritual, the next instruction reminded sisters that 'we cannot reach heaven, except by using earthly things, the Sisters, to gain souls by works of mercy, ought to show themselves willing to render the lowest service to those who are in distress'.[24] Thus visiting often meant attending to the material and as well as health needs of those they called on. Daughter of Charity Soeur Augustine (Catherine) Eyston (1824–1894) went visiting the sick poor with 'a bottle of milk or soup up her sleeve, a big brown-paper parcel of poor clothes in her arms, her apron tucked up at the back and her gamp held firmly in her hand'.[25] Sisters also addressed some grave medical cases whilst visiting and provided basic nursing care which used not only dietetics but also incorporated current understandings of hygiene. Fille de la Croix Noelie Brodesser wrote of her visiting the sick poor with Sister Honorine:

> I often accompanied her to visit the sick. The first time I accompanied her, we visited a girl of 13 who was suffering from Tubercles disease. She had a discharging wound in the neck, and through neglect, the disease had eaten its way into the throat. The poor child was in a sad condition. I was afraid to go near the couch, but Sister Honorine was not. Although the child was in a filthy state, like the good samaritan, she took her in her arms, regardless of the vermin, that was crawling all over her, and the wound had been neglected, the discharge had dried on the poor little body, and made it very sore. She carefully bathed her, and gently dressed the wounds, put clean linen on which she had brought with her and left her consoled and comfortable, nor did she forget the spiritual part. She instructed, and prepared her for first communion, which she made most fervently. The Mother of the child was a poor Shiftless woman, who could not touch her without hurting her, which accounts for the child's neglected condition. Sister Honorine continued to nurse and care for the child, until her death, which took place a year later. I always noticed, when we had a more repulsive and disagreeable case than usual, Sister Honorine always lavished more love and affection on that one.[26]

Of course, this entry was meant as a tribute to Sister Honorine and served, within the congregation, as a tool to edify religious sisters and encourage gentleness and kindness when facing difficult medical cases. But putting these pious intentions aside, it also identifies how nursing knowledge was transmitted as well as what knowledge was necessary for domiciliary nursing. The apprenticeship model was an explicit component of sharing nursing knowledge in nineteenth-century women's congregations. Sister Noelie Brodesser was taught 'practical skills' in the homes of the poor by Sister Honorine. Other congregations noted similar practices. The novices of the Congregation of St Joseph of Peace 'learned what it was to tend the sick-poor by accompanying Mother Evangelista or another professed Sister, on their routine visits to the poor parts of the parish. They went carrying hot food to some poor invalid; or armed with soap and cloths, prepared to wash and lay-out some neglected

---

24   SMG, Rule & Constitutions of the Poor Servants of the Mother of God and the Poor (1892), Chapter XIV.
25   Archives of the Daughters of Charity of St Vincent de Paul, Mill Hill, London, 11–87 1–1 #5, p. 3. The gamp was a commonly used term for an umbrella.
26   Archives of the Filles de la Croix, E/Kersten Maria, Memoir by Sister Noelie Brodesser about Sr Honorine.

corpse.'[27] As the practice of visiting the sick was routine amongst Catholic religious congregations in England, this model of learning, the inexperienced being taught by the experienced, was probably commonplace.

Lectures

Some congregations went further and formalised their training within the congregation. The congregation of the Little Company of Mary founded by Mary Potter (1847–1913) in 1877 operated hospitals in Limerick, Rome and Australia and practiced domiciliary nursing in England.[28] Potter was emphatic that the sisters be medically educated. The first draft of the congregation's 'Rule and Constitutions' instructed that a 'Conference on Nursing' be given 'at a fixed hour in each week by the Rev. Mother or by the Sister Infirmarian under the direction to all the Sisters who may be present in the house'.[29] Thus, Mother M. Philip (Edith) Coleridge (1843–1927), a trained nurse from St George's Hospital, who had entered religious life in 1877 gave lectures on 'practical nursing' at 4pm every weekday.[30] Potter insisted that after each nursing lecture, the sister-nurses would discuss what they had learned.[31] Later, they were questioned about their clinical knowledge to see if 'they have paid attention'.[32] Potter demanded of M. Rose (Mary) Moules, Novice Mistress in Australia: 'Be particular about the Nursing lectures. Make them learn by heart and also give them practical lessons, putting on leeches, going to bed to be poulticed, sheets changed, etc.'[33]

Mother Mary Potter also encouraged lecture series on medical and scientific topics by local doctors. Dr Henry R. Hatherly, a Protestant surgeon on staff at Nottingham Women's Hospital, was co-opted into giving a series of nursing lectures to supplement Mother Philip's 'practical lessons'.[34] His medical lectures were a regular feature in the English motherhouse in Nottingham. In one missal to M. Catherine (Maria) Crocker, Potter notes that 'All at present busy with Nursing Lectures' and that 'Am sorry this is the last lecture of the course. We must try and get Dr Collins now, for a fresh course, especially as

---

27 Ferguson (1983), p. 80.
28 The congregation spread to Ireland, Italy, Malta, Australia and North America by 1900.
29 LCM, 'Original Copy of the First Draft on the Rule Prepared by Bishop Bagshawe', p. 2.
30 LCM, 14/12, M. Hilda, 'Some Memories of Mary Potter' (1957), pp. 55–56; 15/8 Place of Springs (1977), p. 19.
31 LCM, Conferences 'M', p. 27.
32 LCM, Conferences 'Q', 'Early Customs and Directions', p. 2.
33 LCM, Book I, Undated letter from Mary Potter to M. Rose (Mary) Moules, p. 107.
34 LCM, 14/12, M. Hilda, 'Some Memories of Mary Potter' (1957), p. 57; Hatherly was Mary Potter's personal doctor, a Member of the Royal College of Surgeons (MRCS England 1864) and a Licentiate of the Royal College of Physicians (LRCP Edinburgh 1867). He was on staff at the Women's Hospital in Nottingham and was a member of the Medico-Chirurgical Society. I am grateful to Geraldine O'Driscoll of The Royal College of Surgeons of England for clarifying information about Dr Hatherly's medical credentials.

we have several nurses coming.'[35] Potter wrote to Sister Magdalen (Elizabeth) Bryan (1833–1898):

> Do have the Nursing Lectures regularly, and have a lecture from a Doctor when you can get one. There is quite a regular enquiry going on about our training, and we say in England they have nursing lectures from Doctors, etc., but really Mother, the lectures must be experimental: Can they put a leech on?
> Can they compress?
> Give injections.
> Draw water.
> Feel the pulse and not the respirations.
> Do they without exception keep the Report.[36]

The content of these 'experimental' lectures, as we'll explore in the last section of this essay, is consistent with nineteenth-century nurse training practices.

Mary Potter linked the importance of nurse education with vocation. She urged her sisters to 'be prepared for your duties to the sick and dying, for without that you would dishonour instead of honouring our Lady. This we soon discovered, and now have Doctors of our own especially appointed to train the Sisters.'[37]

While patient care was an important means in and of itself, Potter felt compelled to have her sisters considered 'trained nurses' by those outside Catholic circles. Criticisms were waged against the quality of medical care in Catholic institutions. Speaking generally on convent care in Rome, one anonymous contributor to *The British Medical Journal* noted that there was a paucity of institutions where English patients could obtain 'care and skilled nursing'. He dismissed the nursing done by 'the good sisters' who were 'untrained, and display some jealousy of trained interference'.[38] Physician and Surgeon John J. Eyre, responding to this claim in the next issue of the *The British Medical Journal*, retorted that though the Little Company of Mary had at one time sisters with 'no regular hospital training, but for all that they were not by any means incompetent nurses. Now, however, almost all of them are hospital trained and certificated nurses.'[39] By 1899, when this was written, much of the training of the Little Company of Mary nurses was obtained at the hospital the congregation opened in Milford, County Limerick, Ireland. Here, Irish and English sisters were trained on the wards from 1888. This nursing education, however, was fairly inconsistent in the early years of the hospital, and Dr John F. Devane, Chief Physician eventually delivered a regular series of lectures on anatomy, physiology, medicine and surgery.[40]

---

35   LCM, Book H, Letter from Mary Potter to M. Catherine (Maria) Crocker dated Nativity Eve, p. 63.
36   LCM, Book E, Undated letter from Mary Potter to M. Magdalen (Elizabeth) Bryan.
37   LCM, Conferences 'R', p. 24.
38   *The British Medical Journal* (1899), p. 1050.
39   Eyre (1899), p. 1194. The Little Company of Mary was often referred to as the English Nursing Sisters.
40   Devane (1970), pp. 42, 50, 71–72, 99. John F. Devane was a Fellow of the Royal College of Surgeons and obtained his medical degree from the National University of Ireland. He

Sisters were also given lectures by doctors on staff in other congregation hospitals including Providence Free Hospital in St Helens and St John and St Elizabeth's Hospital in London.[41] When the Sisters of Mercy from Bermondsey returned from the Crimea, they were immediately asked to open and manage London's first post-reformation Catholic hospital, St John and St Elizabeth. They used the knowledge gained from their experience as military nurses and trained sister-nurses on the wards of the hospital. By 1898, as nursing knowledge evolved, another level of nursing education was deemed necessary and Dr Cahill was asked to deliver a series of eighteen lectures to the sister-nurses.[42] In 1903, the lecture series was expanded to include surgical lectures given as the doctors and sisters went around the wards.[43]

While many questions remain unanswered about the quality of the nurse training itself, the congregations discussed were serious about nursing knowledge and their sister-nurses obtaining both a practical and in some cases, a medicalised and scientific education. Knowledge was obtained through European convent networks where English sister-nurses from congregations obtained medical skills targeted to the specific needs of the poor in their institutions. The apprenticeship model was also used to train nurse-sisters; it was ubiquitous within religious congregations as it was an efficient and inexpensive means of teaching practical skills and knowledge. For some congregations, a series of lectures taught by nurses or doctors introduced both practical skills and medical knowledge to nursing sisters. What still remains to be addressed however was whether the content of the training being disseminated to nursing sisters was congruent with nursing knowledge being obtained outside convent networks.

Nineteenth-century nursing knowledge

The traditional whiggish history of nursing has developed teleologically, heralding the heroic journey towards formal education, professionalisation and the implementation of nursing registration as the successful endgoal. Throughout this historiography, informal means of obtaining knowledge were summarily dismissed while formal means were proclaimed as important evidence of professionalisation. As this next section shall show, the general means of obtaining nursing knowledge in late nineteenth-century England remained linked to 'practical training' and the quality of 'trained nurses' varied.

Florence Nightingale's contribution to nursing knowledge was the separation of the doctor's responsibility, the patient's body, from the nurse's respon-

was Senior House Physician in Mater Misericordiae Hospital in Dublin (the largest teaching hospital in Ireland) before he joined St John's Hospital.

41 SMG, III/SH/BOY 22 Report Providence Free Hospital (1900), p. 15.
42 LMA, SC/PPS/093 26.1, Hospital of St John and St Elizabeth Annual Report (1898), pp. 12–13.
43 Nursing by the Sisters of Mercy. In: The Hospital (3 October 1903).

sibility, the patient's environment. Her rejection of germ theory, and all-consuming embrace of hygiene, allowed the focus of nursing knowledge to veer towards clinical practice. This holistic view bound the physical and the moral, and was reflected in Nightingale's expectation that nurses be 'fundamentally moral'. Charles Rosenberg calls the hospital a 'moral universe' where nurses brought order and cleanliness in accordance with Nightingale's nursing dictates. Her understanding of disease aetiology hinged on the connections between human behaviour, human environment and human health. Thus the physical attributes of filth embodied an 'absolute moral otherness'.[44] She balanced the tensions between theory and practice by acknowledging that nurses needed to absorb enough medical and scientific knowledge in order to understand the instructions of physicians. Risjord calls this the 'theory-practice gap' where medical knowledge was translated into clinical practice.[45] This medical and scientific knowledge was only part of the nurse's knowledge, the crux of their knowledge base, according to Nightingale was learned through clinical practice.

An important body of nursing knowledge was articulated in Florence Nightingale's influential list of nurse skills and duties, which can be divided into the following categories:

• hygiene: helping patients (moving, changing, personal cleanliness, feeding, keeping warm or cool, preventing and dressing bed-sores); bandaging (making bandages, rollers, lining of splints); making beds; keeping wards fresh; cleanliness of utensils
• dietetics: sick cooking (gruel, arrowroot, egg flip, pudding, drinks)
• therapeutics: dressings (blisters, burns, sores, wounds, fomentations, poultices, minor dressings); applying leeches; enemas; management of trusses and uterine appliances; rubbing; waiting on operations
• observation: management of convalescents; observations (secretions, expectorations, pain, skin, appetite, intelligence, breathing, sleep, state of wounds, eruptions, formations of matter, effect of diet, stimulants and medicines, signs of approaching death)[46]

By organising the nurse skills and duties in this way, one can see the broad skills that were important to nineteenth-century nursing knowledge. Carol Helmstadter has argued that there were other influences on nursing knowledge. She argues that 'new medicine' caused a shift in therapeutics mid-century. Nursing practice became more specialised as hygiene became an important component of nursing knowledge and thus apparently mundane tasks such as the making and washing of dressings took on a clinical value deriving from new understandings of clinical medicine. Special diets and stimulants replaced the depleting remedies of bleeding, purging, vomiting and blistering.

---

44   Rosenberg (1979), pp. 122–126.
45   Risjord (2010), pp. 6–8.
46   Parliamentary Papers (henceforth PP) (1890), p. 616, Appendix.

Medical understandings led to the promulgation of continuous rather than intermittent patient care.[47]

Numerous other historians have examined nurse duties and skills and linked them to medical and scientific understandings of the nineteenth century. At a time when specialty pharmaceuticals such as intravenous therapies were unavailable, the use of special diets and stimulants can be transformed into twenty-first century 'nutritional and fluid management'. The act of cleaning a patient's body could be a 'prescribed intervention' if the patient had a fever.[48] Bathing, poultices, plasters, bindings were required as a measure of clinical competence. Erysipelas was a common skin ailment in hospitals as was general debility and unhealed ulcers; hospital treatment for these conditions was the seemingly unsophisticated bed rest and diet. Bed rest, though sounding simplistic, is still a prescribed medical treatment that involves a period of continuous recumbence.[49] The observation and recording of pulses, temperatures, etc. were a means to understanding disease processes. Today, these are often monitored using biophysical or physiological equipment such as sphygmomanometer (blood pressure meter), pulse oximeter (measures oxygen saturation of a patient's blood) or cardiac output monitors (volume of blood being pumped by the heart). Surgical treatment became more frequent in twentieth-century hospitals and new skills were needed for this but nineteenth-century therapeutics remained factors in the aftercare of surgical patients.[50] Dingwall and Allen as well as Nelson and Gordon claim that what today is seen as 'caring' nursing practice was as advanced as the science of the times.[51] Jose Harris has argued that improvements in medical care were due more to the 'better practical management of patients' than to the advances of bacteriology and pharmacology. Thus, these therapeutic tasks required new skills that were part of the developing medical knowledge of the nineteenth century.[52]

These therapeutic 'practical skills' were the ones learned by Catholic sister-nurses whether being trained by their European counter-parts or by other sister-nurses through the apprenticeship system. In printed material, Florence Nightingale's dictums on cleanliness held resonance in Catholic hospital spaces. The 'Rule and Constitutions' of the Poor Servants instructed sister-nurses that 'they must spare no labour to secure order and cleanliness in all things' and that 'They must be intelligent, attentive and obedient to all the doctor says, never opposing his wishes.' Daughter of Charity Soeur Augustine used dietetics to nurse her patients. The Poor Servants learned skills in comforting and feeding the sick poor from the Augustinians. Fille de la Croix Noe-

---

47 Helmstadter (2002), pp. 325–326.
48 Dingwall/Allen (2001), p. 67.
49 For the debates of the efficacy of bedrest over early ambulation see Allen/Glasziou/Del Mar (1999).
50 Dingwall/Allen (2001), p. 67.
51 Nelson/Gordon (2004), pp. 258–259; Dingwall/Allen (2001).
52 Harris (1993), p. 56.

lie Brodesser was skilled in bathing the patient and dressing wounds. Mary Potter expected the Little Company's nursing sisters to be knowledgable in applying leeches, compresses, giving injections, observing pulse and respirations and reporting on their observations. The Poor Servants learned dispensary skills. Lectures in anatomy, physiology, medicine and surgery were delivered to the sisters of the Little Company of Mary, the Sisters of Mercy and the Poor Servants of the Mother of God.

The important question as to the 'quality' of nurse training and patient care is much more difficult to answer. In the nineteenth century, nurse training was not uniform. Certificated 'trained nurses' were not consistently trained or tested. And many practicing nurses remained uncertificated. Medical lectures could be regular or intermittent and were dependent on the availability of physicians. Nurses with certificates from specialist hospitals or small cottage hospitals may not have had the same exposure to the variety of medical cases as had nurses in large metropolitan hospitals. There were disagreements as to how much and what kind of training was needed for a 'trained nurse'. On 7 July 1890, Eva Lückes, then matron at the London Hospital, went before the Select Committee on Metropolitan Hospitals to discuss current nursing practices. In identifying what constituted a 'trained nurse', Lückes explained to the committee that she believed a year's training was all that was needed for a nurse to be 'technically trained' and noted that some probationers became sisters before they had their nursing certificates.[53] Probationer nurses were the majority of the staff in most hospitals and though medical and scientific training may have been a part of their education, more common were the long hours on the ward learning through clinical practice. Lückes also noted that nursing knowledge was primarily obtained on the ward.[54] Lückes was referring to the apprenticeship model of nurse training which nurse historian Ann Bradshaw has argued was 'remodelled and rearticulated' by Florence Nightingale to fit a Protestant nursing culture.[55] This feature of nurse education was ubiquitous throughout nineteenth-century England.

What was unique about Catholic nurse training was the temporal needs of the patient were explicitly weaved into the spiritual. The Sister of the Little Company of Mary was instructed that:

> the soul is her one principle work … It will be this Sister's special charge. She must be a mother to that soul and not cease her continual inward prayer in all the outward works she performs for the sufferer. They need not distract her. In washing the sick person she may be praying that the soul likewise may be cleansed from the slightest stain of sin. In giving food the sister can be praying that her charge may be strengthened by the Bread of Life and so on. The Sister may not consider it is a light duty she has undertaken, but a very solemn and serious one.[56]

---

53 PP (1890), p. 378, paragraph 6499; p. 390, paragraphs 6611–6613.
54 PP (1890), p. 375, paragraph 6457.
55 Bradshaw (2001), p. 1.
56 LCM, Conferences 'M', Mary Potter, 'Rules Regarding Novices in the Future State of Our Institute' (1876), p. 6.

This link between nursing the body and the salvation of the soul was imbricated in a religious sister's vocation.

Conclusion

In terms of nursing knowledge, Catholic women religious did not emphasise altering or contributing specific knowledge to the nursing curriculum; their focus was on spiritual and temporal care. They aimed for a more holistic practice that enabled the cure of the body and soul. This centred not only on the patient's medical requirements, but also emotional and spiritual requirements. Their focus on patients with chronic conditions or in need of long-term care meant that therapeutic practices and medical skills, espoused by Florence Nightingale and medical clinicians of the time, that tended towards hygiene, dietetics and therapeutics were most beneficial for patients in Catholic institutions. By the nature of their health care needs, patient cohorts influenced the way the nursing sisters worked and were trained. Many of the poor in need of medical care were not treated in the voluntary hospitals which for most of the nineteenth century operated to meet the needs of medical science and provided a practical training ground for physicians.

Catholic health care institutions developed from the interplay of a variety of factors: funding, competition, the philanthropic objects of the religious congregation, the perceived needs of a locality and the spectre of anti-catholicism, both real and imagined. These patient cohorts and Catholic understanding of faith and healing influenced the ways in which health knowledge was transmitted. Health knowledge was transmitted both formally and informally, both internationally and locally, via a variety of agents. In the developing environment of nurse professionalisation, informal methods of giving, receiving and utilising nursing knowledge have often been seen as inadequate. Yet, for all nurse trainees, the corpus of nursing knowledge remained undefined and the term 'trained nurse' did not assume a consistent level of knowledge or training in the late nineteenth century. Informal networks of knowledge, like those of Catholic religious sisters, transmitted knowledge that was congruent with the medical knowledge of the time. This shared knowledge was real knowledge based on practical experience and should not be dismissed.

Bibliography

Allen, Chris; Glasziou, Paul; Del Mar, Chris: Bed rest: a potentially harmful treatment needing more careful evaluation. In: The Lancet 354 (1999), pp. 1229–1234.

Baly, Monica E.: Nursing and Social Change. London; New York 1973.

Bradshaw, Ann: The Nurse Apprentice, 1860–1977. Aldershot 2001.

Burdett, Henry C.: Burdett's Hospital Annual and Year Book of Philanthropy. London 1901.

The Catholic Directory, ecclesiastical register, and almanac. London 1900.

Devane, John F.: A History of St John's Hospital, Limerick. Dublin 1970.

Devas, Francis Charles: Mother Mary Magdalen of the Sacred Heart (Fanny Margaret Tay-
    lor): Foundress of the Poor Servants of the Mother of God 1832–1900. London 1927.
Dingwall, Robert; Allen, Davina: The implications of healthcare reforms for the profession of
    nursing. In: Nursing Inquiry 8 (2001), pp. 64–74.
Dingwall, Robert; Rafferty, Anne Marie; Webster, Charles: An Introduction to the Social His-
    tory of Nursing. London 1988.
Eyre, John: Nursing Homes in Rome. In: The British Medical Journal 1 (1899), issue 2002,
    p. 1193–1194.
Ferguson, Catherine: Sisters of St Joseph of Peace: History of the Sacred Heart Province,
    1884–1984. Rearsby 1983.
Green, Teresa: The English Sisters of Mercy in the Crimean War. In: History of Nursing Soci-
    ety Journal 5 (1994/95), no. 3, pp. 119–127.
Harris, Jose: Private Lives, Public Spirit: Britain 1870–1914. Oxford 1993.
Helmstadter, Carol: Early Nursing Reform in Nineteenth-Century London: A Doctor-Driven
    Phenomenon. In: Medical History 46 (2002), pp. 325–350.
Jones, Colin: Sisters of Charity and the Ailing Poor. In: Social History of Medicine 2 (1989),
    no. 3, pp. 339–348.
Jones, Colin: The Charitable Imperative: Hospitals and Nursing in Ancien Regime and Revo-
    lutionary France. London 1989.
Maggs, Christopher: The Origin of General Nursing. London 1983.
Mangion, Carmen: Contested Identities: Catholic Women Religious in nineteenth-century
    England and Wales. Manchester 2008.
Nelson, Sioban; Gordon, Suzanne: The rhetoric of rupture: Nursing as a practice with a his-
    tory? In: Nursing Outlook 52 (2004), no. 5, pp. 255–261.
Nelson, Sioban: Say Little, Do Much: Nurses, Nuns, and Hospitals in the Nineteenth Century.
    Philadelphia 2001.
Parliamentary Papers (1890), paper no. 392. Report from the Select Committee of the House
    of Lords on metropolitan hospitals, &c.; together with the proceedings of the committee,
    minutes of evidence, and appendix.
Risjord, Mark: Nursing Knowledge: Science, Practice, and Philosophy. Chichester 2010.
Rosenberg, Charles E.: Florence Nightingale on Contagion: The Hospital as Moral Universe.
    In: Rosenberg, Charles E. (ed.): Healing and History: Essays for George Rosen. New York;
    Folkestone 1979, pp. 116–136.
Seymer, Lucy R.: Florence Nightingale's Nurses. The Nightingale Training School, 1860–
    1960. London 1960.
Wildman, Stuart: The Development of Nurse Training in Birmingham Teaching Hospitals,
    1869–1957. In: International History of Nursing Journal 7 (2003), pp. 56–65.
Woodward, John: To Do the Sick No Harm: A Study of the British Voluntary Hospital System
    to 1875. London 1974.

"Local Missionaries": Community deaconesses in early nineteenth-century health care[*]

Karen Nolte

Introduction

The hygiene movement, which had started around 1800, promoted three virtues in particular: neatness, cleanliness and morality. The target of such attempts to create a health discipline was mainly the urban proletariat.[1] As Ute Frevert has emphasized, women were the recipients and the agents of these middle class endeavors to improve hygiene.[2] The following article deals with a group of female protagonists involved in the bourgeois hygiene and health education which has been so far largely ignored by the scholarship: Since the 1840s the school for deaconesses in Kaiserswerth near Düsseldorf sent young women into poor urban neighborhoods. These women had been systematically trained as nurses and guardians of the poor. The founder of the school, the Lutheran pastor Theodor Fliedner, employed deaconesses to fight disease, poverty and impiety and thus reacted to the urgent 'social issue' that had arisen already during the first half of the 19th century. The driving forces of the 'inner mission' drew a direct causal link between the increasing impiety and the dramatic pauperization of the working classes. For that reason, their attempts to decrease material poverty were equal to their efforts to save the souls of the poor. While Frevert mentions the "missionary eagerness" of the ladies who worked as educators and guardians in the impoverished neighborhoods in the nineteenth century, she does not analyze the religious dimension of the educational program these middle class women and nurses embraced.[3]

The following paper addresses precisely the specific notions and practices of hygiene and health care that these protestant community nurses embraced.

In her study on collective identities ("Kollektive Identitäten") of the deaconesses in Kaiserswerth, Silke Köser analyzes the extraordinary role that the cleanliness drill played during the deaconesses' training in Kaiserswerth.[4] She draws on the work of ethnologist Mary Douglas on "Purity and Danger" and

---

[*] This article is part of the research project "Wege zu einer Alltagsgeschichte der Ethik. Vom Umgang mit Schwerkranken (1500–1800)" (Ways to an Everyday History of Ethics. About the Interaction with the Critically Ill) supported by the Fritz Thyssen Foundation and headed by Prof. Dr. Dr. Michael Stolberg. Translator: Ulrike Nichols.

1 On bourgeois concepts of hygiene and during the 19th century: Labisch (1992), pp. 111–141; Sarasin (2001); Löneke/Spieker (1996).
2 See Frevert (1984); Frevert (1985).
3 On the female philanthropy and expansion of bourgeois concepts of hygiene in Britain's "working class" see also Bashford (1998).
4 See Köser (2006), pp. 303–306.

stresses that dirt was understood to be synonymous with disorder.[5] Hence cleaning had to be regarded as a positive effort to bring order back into one's life. Emphasizing the value of cleanliness for the deaconesses' self-image, the institution drew on nineteenth century bourgeois concepts of hygiene. These ideals used cleanliness and order as metaphors for ethical and moral integrity. A deaconess' crucial quality was her sexual abstinence. Along with Mary Douglas, Köser argues that regular physical washing procedures and cleaning were to keep the "moral demand for cleanliness" present in the nurses' minds.[6]

Using the deaconesses' everyday reports, I will illustrate in the following that the nurses also linked piety, that is, a 'healthy' condition of the soul, to bourgeois concepts of hygiene. By contrast, their views of dirt, disease, poverty and impiety were inextricably connected.

My sources are letters that deaconesses sent to the directors (a couple consisting of husband and wife) of the mother house in Kaiserswerth, in which they reported on their work and experiences with their patients in the community. If one reads between the lines, these sources from the nurses' everyday life also grant a glimpse into the life of the people living in the poor neighborhood and their responses to the "charitable siege"[7] on which the Christian nurses had embarked.

The deaconesses of Kaiserswerth and their letters

Nursing care in nineteenth century Germany was greatly influenced by the motherhouse system. At that time, the motherhouses offered one of few opportunities for unmarried women for acquiring sound professional training and living respectable lives outside marriage or their parents' home. In return for lifelong employment and being taken care of in their old age, the sisters were expected to devote their lives to the service of the sister community. The motherhouse assumed the function of parental care and control for the young women who thus became 'daughters' in these substitute families. For example, the sisters could be relocated to a new workplace by the motherhouses at any time, even against their will.[8] The successful motherhouse system was also adopted by secular nursing organizations such as the German Red Cross. In the late nineteenth century, alongside the sisters bound to a motherhouse, about 22% of nurses worked as self-employed private care nurses under precarious conditions.[9] They were not covered in case of sickness nor were they

---

5   See Douglas (1966).
6   See Köser (2006), p. 305.
7   Frevert (1985).
8   See Kreutzer (2005), pp. 34–36.
9   According to vocational statistics of the Kaiserliches Gesundheitsamt (Imperial Health Office) of 1876, nurses belonging to a religious community made up 61.6% of all nurses; of these, 38.5% were Catholic and 23.1% Protestant. 16.1% of the nurses belonged to a secular association, and 22.3% were self-employed, see Seidler/Leven (2003), p. 225.

entitled to old-age insurance or pension.[10] Facilitated by the availability of excellent historical records, the following study focuses on the institution for deaconesses in Kaiserswerth which was very influential in the historical development of nursing care in Germany.

The archives of the Fliedner-Kulturstiftung (Fliedner Culture Foundation) in Kaiserswerth near Düsseldorf hold a comprehensive inventory of letters sent on a regular basis by the nurses who were dispatched by the deaconess motherhouse to hospitals, parish or private nursing care all over the German Reich. The letters were addressed to the directing pastor and directing sister of the motherhouse[11] and contained reports about the nurses' work and their experiences at their location[12].

In the training of the deaconesses of Kaiserswerth the nursing of the soul – caring for the welfare of the soul of the sick person – was just as important as nursing the sick body.[13] After finishing their training in the motherhouse, the deaconesses were sent out to hospitals and into parish and private care in many German cities. The founder of the first German deaconess motherhouses, Theodor Fliedner (1800–1864), originally intended this training for daughters of the educated middle class – in particular daughters of pastors and doctors. Up to that point, nursing had been a profession that almost exclusively attracted women and men of the lower social classes which meant that its standing in society was comparable to a servant's position. For this reason, at first mostly young women of the lower middle class and from farming families were willing to become deaconesses. It was not until the second half of the nineteenth century that more and more women from the upper middle class joined the deaconess institutions and first held leading positions in nursing such as that of directing sister.[14]

In the tradition of the paternalistic-familial leadership model created by Theodor Fliedner, the directing pastor and the directing sister of the deaconess motherhouse in Kaiserswerth saw themselves not simply as the deaconesses' superiors. Rather, they saw themselves as substitute "parents" for the young women who needed to supervise "their" deaconesses with love and strictness. The deaconesses actually addressed the directors as "dear parents", "dear mother" and "dear father" in their letters and entrusted to them their problems great and small, everyday experiences and inner questions of faith.

---

10 See Seidler/Leven (2003), pp. 223–228.
11 Theodor Fliedner based his community of deaconesses on the model of the Order of the Sisters of Mercy and adopted from them the concept of the motherhouse in the sense that it was a place of origin for the community. According to this concept, the motherhouse was and is the place where the deaconesses were trained and from where they were sent to their work.
12 Archives of the Fliedner-Kulturstiftung in Kaiserswerth/Düsseldorf (hereafter FSAK), Letters from Sisters.
13 At first, the training was brief: It lasted only two months and only gradually increased in length.
14 See Schmidt (1998), pp. 161–216; Felgentreff (1998), pp. 22–23.

The letters of the deaconesses and probationary nurses show very clearly how much the writers were trying to achieve the ideal image of a deaconess and thus to fulfill the expectations of the directors.[15] The official regulations – which specified their communal living and working in the deaconess community as well as Christian and civic virtues – were to be taken to heart, mainly on the basis of the catalogue of "questions for introspection" designed by Theodor Fliedner. These questions were aimed at fortifying the young women's faith and Christian demeanor and at providing a structure for the daily introspection that was also a subject in the letters.[16] On occasion, extracts of selected letters were published in the in-house magazine *Der Armen- und Krankenfreund* ("Friend of the Poor and Sick") [17] to set an example for other deaconesses. It must be assumed that this influenced the writing behavior of the deaconesses. Thus, these letters are, on the one hand, suited as studies of how the deaconesses saw themselves and were expected to see themselves measuring up to an ideal as nurses and in their relation to the sick. It is evident from the letters that the writers tried to choose a superior style to live up to the educated upper class writing style expected of them; on the other hand, an obvious clumsiness in their phrasing and a large number of orthographic and grammatical errors document that the deaconesses – who into the late nineteenth century mostly came from rural farming families – did not have the necessary education. The idiosyncratic writing style is also an important expression of each single writer's personality. In private and parish nursing, the letters were an important social contact with a familiar partner for the young sisters who might be working alone in unfamiliar surroundings. Hence, the letters also served to help the writers deal with their experiences and conflicts.

The different functions of the letters lead to inconsistencies in these self-testimonials as a result of numerous expectations; these inconsistencies occurred every time the writers unconsciously crossed the lines dictated by an inner self-censorship, in sub-clauses or marginal remarks.

Dirt, faithlessness, disease and poverty

The reports of a nurse from the "Medical Course" on trial at the institution for deaconesses in Kaiserswerth in 1850[18] reveal that two standard volumes, written by the doctors Carl Emil Gedike (1797–1867) and Johann Friedrich Dieffenbach (1792–1847)[19] respectively, were crucial for the training in physical care. Unlike contemporary manuals on nursing care[20], the manual used in

---

15   See Köser (2006).
16   Köser (2006), pp. 217–219.
17   The magazines are also kept in the FSAK.
18   See FSAK, Medicinischer Cursus, Sign.: Rep II:Fd.
19   Both doctors were directors of the school for nurses at the Charité-Hospital in Berlin.
20   Cf. also Krügelstein (1807). Franz Christian Karl Krügelstein (1779–1864) was a country doctor in Ohrdruf near Gotha.

Kaiserswerth specifies – under the heading "Qualities of a Good Nurse" – religious purity as the first and foremost requirement of a nurse. Furthermore, this was strictly differentiated from "outer qualities" such as "neatness and cleanliness". In the "House Rules and Service Regulations for Deaconesses" religious and moral "purity" is emphasized as a crucial condition for the admission into the community of deaconesses: "Fallen individuals will not be admitted even if they have changed for the better."[21] Yet for the Christian nursing care "outer cleanliness" was also crucial: Nurses on probation and deaconesses were supposed to internalize the cleanliness necessary for caring through "questions for introspection", as hygiene was apparently not yet seen as a requirement for health.[22]

Fliedner emphasized that due to their gender, deaconesses were especially suited to perform the "hygiene training" in lower class families.

> A deacon could never teach a housewife how to keep the house clean and orderly, how to wash children that are running around, wild and filthy and in ragged clothes, how to mend their clothes and darn their socks – or those of the husband, or show how the housewife, in addition to the housework, could earn an extra income with knitting, sewing, and spinning. However, a one-off visit by a pious, well meaning lady alone could not have a very beneficial effect on housewives and adult daughters, because the effort must not be a singular but a sustained one.[23]

Simultaneously, he differentiates here between the ongoing teachings in hygiene through trained nurses and the activities of the bourgeois female philanthropists who, according to him, were supposed to work merely as assistants of community deaconesses.[24]

"Outer" cleanliness is mentioned first in the medical manuals under the headings of the qualities necessary for a nurse (either male or female). The repeated emphasis that good nurses would stand out because of their cleanliness and orderliness, points to the assumption that, in contrast to the deaconesses, an untrained paid careworker was dirty and messy. Similarly, in the UK, it was the "new nurse" with a middle class background who was supposed to teach "working class" people cleanliness as an important measure to prevent diseases. She was juxtaposed to the "old nurse" who was portrayed as dirty and untidy, had a tendency to drink and was prone to moral failures.[25] For the nurses who had received a careful Christian-moral training in Kaiserswerth, cleanliness was a crucial feature of distinction from the untrained paid careworkers who worked in most hospitals. Walter Klein's study on the work performed by the Kaiserswerth deaconesses in the citizens' hospital in Saarbrücken supports this notion: Klein describes how, in the 1840s, the deaconess

---

21 FSAK, Haus-Ordnung und Dienst-Anweisung für die Diakonissen (House Rules and Service Regulations for Deaconesses), Kaiserswerth 1852, p. 10, Sign.: I Rep. II: Fc1.
22 See Selbstprüfungsfragen (1855), p. 11.
23 Fliedner (1860), p. 74.
24 Fliedner (1860), p. 74.
25 See Bashford (1998). In England, especially Florence Nightingale had shaped ideas of cleanliness in health care, cf. Nightingale (1860).

moved into the hospital and immediately addressed the carelessness of the careworkers on site; neglect which they saw rooted mainly in the "dirt, grease and lice" that they had seen in the wards.[26] Klein's sources stem from the time when the institution for deaconesses was founded in Kaiserswerth and they suggest that the thorough cleaning that happened after the deaconesses had moved into the hospital in Saarbrücken also bore the ritual character referred to by Douglas. Thus, the nurses reported to the motherhouse that they had "pulled" the citizens' hospital "out of the dirt".

The letters that I will subsequently analyze also date from the time when the Kaiserswerth institution opened. In these letters the nurses described their tasks and activities: The deaconesses were first sent into impoverished urban neighborhoods during the 1840s to care for sick people and to fight the material and spiritual poverty of these patients. To ease material poverty, the patients were to be provided with jobs and an income. The deaconesses supplied the poor people with some bare necessities for life, bringing them goods "collected" from richer community members, which meant that they had gone begging from door to door for the poor. The deaconesses were thus to remind the community members of their Christian duty to love their neighbors.[27] The deaconesses described the practice of collecting these goods as time-consuming and humiliating.[28] The nurses coordinated the help from the various welfare organizations on site to prevent instances of double or even multiple support and thus their work was essential for the communal welfare for the poor.

The spiritual condition of the poor patients, the soul care, was important for the community deaconesses. They believed that poverty and disease were causally linked to impiety and sin and concluded that the impoverished patients' spiritual purification, the healing of the soul, was just as important as physical care for the sick bodies and material care against poverty. Accordingly, bringing the patients back to faith was crucial for the entire healing process. At the same time, a righteous and pious way of life was seen as an important condition for staying healthy. For that reason the deaconesses also visited "healthy" families in impoverished areas, seeking to elevate their "soul status" to bring the "inner, secret corruption" – of which the pastors were not even aware – "to the light of day".[29] The idea was that the deaconesses who themselves had lower class backgrounds found easier access to the souls of the poor than the pastors who came from the educated middle class.

---

26 Cf. Klein (2002), p. 96.
27 See FSAK, Haus-Ordnung und Dienst-Anweisung für die Diakonissen in der Diakonissen-Anstalt zu Kaiserswerth 1852 (House Rules and Service Regulations for Deaconesses in Kaiserswerth 1852), Sign.: Gr.Fl. IV i 3², p. 76.
28 See FSAK, Cleve, Letters from Nurses 1845–1854, Sign.: 1337, Dorothee Haube, 11.2.1853. Sister Dorothee wrote to the principal couple that she lost a lot of time due to her "running around with the collection box".
29 See Fliedner (1860), p. 73.

During the first house calls, the encounters with the poor families exceeded the deaconesses' worst expectations with regard to both the state of mind as well as material conditions. Sister Elisabeth reports from Elberfeld in 1849:

> I would never have thought that you could find such misery in a famous Christian town like this. It would not be too much if ten community deaconesses were to work here. They would surely find enough work, as there are houses where eight or ten families live together, of which one is more depraved than the next [...] Well, now you give these nice people everything they ask for. Oh – then you are sweet and kind, but if you bring a Bible instead and point out their sins to them – then, they immediately say that if that was all you had come for you could just as well stay away. They had known for some time that they were sinners.[30]

Finally, Sister Elisabeth criticized that the pastors mainly left it to the community deaconesses to visit the poor: "I think the situation would be different if the pastors visited the poor and sick people more frequently but they don't know them. Dear Pastor, people cannot reform themselves if the Lord does not do it but He is accomplishing his work also with mankind as His tool."[31]

The writings of the deaconesses reveal the close religious link that was drawn to cleanliness and purity, expressing the intrinsic connection between sin, faithlessness and dirt.[32] A report from 1880 summarizes this connection describing the dirt and disorder in the houses of the poor:

> We have to visit more than 60 poor families here. It is unbelievable what poverty and misery you often find here: the parents untidy and devoted to the bottle. The children are running around, barely wearing essential clothing, they have no proper bed other than old dirty rags. It is rarely just one of the parents who is responsible for such degradation. It is so obvious here that sin is the corruption of the people.[33]

After stepping into the houses of the poor for the first time, the deaconesses thoroughly cleaned the premises and provided the inhabitants with clean underwear. The extent to which this cleaning can also be seen as a ritual cleansing as described by Mary Douglas, is revealed by the published report of a deaconess who came into a household where previously a catholic Sister of Mercy had been in charge of the care. The Kaiserswerth journal *Friend of the Poor and Sick* reports on the deaconess visiting this family as follows: "She finds them in complete dirt and disorder and her first activity is to make the bed and tidy up the room."[34] The "wrong faith" of the catholic sister is also associated with dirt and disorder which had to be removed immediately. In addition, the soul of the severely ill was in "disorder" as the Catholic nurse was assumed to have caused "horrible fears" in the patient when she was not willing to persuade her protestant children and husband to convert to the Catholic faith.

---

30 FSAK, Elberfeld, Letters of the Sisters 1846–1862, Sign.: 1787, Elisabeth Born, 4.7.1849.
31 FSAK, Elberfeld, Letters of the Sisters 1846–1862, Sign.: 1787, Elisabeth Born, 4.7.1849.
32 The sources Klein cites also reveal how closely the deaconesses linked outer and inner cleanliness and purity: Klein (2002), pp. 96–97.
33 Disselhoff (1880), p. 59.
34 Fliedner (1860), p. 86.

Sister Dorothee reported in 1852 about her first visit to a family in the village of Cleve:

> When I first visited, the woman sat there without a shirt on and within the most horrible dirt [...]. I went there often, organized work for them but also wanted it to be clean there. Since the woman was sickly and the daughter seemed to be a bit out of her senses, I asked them to bring me their dirty laundry every Monday and pick up their clean clothes every Saturday.[35]

The woman declined the deaconess's offer. Presumably she was too embarrassed to allow the sister a glimpse into her most intimate areas and literally have a stranger (from the public) wash her dirty laundry. After that, the deaconess insisted on teaching the family cleanliness: "[...] I wanted to give her soap so that she would not have an excuse for her dirt. But no, they rather get eaten alive by lice than wash themselves."[36] This story is another example for the persistence with which the deaconesses fulfilled their task of serving as health advisers and teachers. The mentioning of the infestation with vermin is striking at this point. The lice serve as a metaphor for the dirt and hence the patient's squalidness. Another report by a community deaconess that was published in 1860 describes how a sinful alcoholic had to be taken to the city hospital regularly "so that he could be cleaned off the vermin". The issue of "vermin" had entered the public discourse as a social problem around 1840; "infestation with vermin" was linked to a social behavior that went against the bourgeois norms.[37] Sister Dorothee's report about another patient makes the link between disorder, dirt and impiety explicit. The critically ill woman had initially refused the deaconess's aid since she could not get physical care without Christian lessons. Dorothee indignantly reported what this "unmarried person" was supposed to have said to a third person after the deaconess's visit: "I [sister Dorothee] could talk. The dear Lord of whom I was talking was on vacation. Those who relied on him were betrayed, and whatever else she had to say [...]."[38] Later the patient's health deteriorated so significantly that she felt forced to accept the deaconess's help. Sister Dorothee very vividly described the misery around that woman which seemed to reflect her spiritual situation, the "state of her soul".

> Glowing with fever she was sitting erect in her bedstead. There was no bed, no sack of straw, indeed, not even straw. She did not wear a shirt and had merely draped an old dress around her. On her back she had a huge abscess which the doctor called a plague-spot [...] She also had a ten-year old child whom lice were about to carry away.[39]

Again the infestation with vermin is heavily emphasized. Dorothee pointed out the connection between severe illness and social adversity that came with the dirt which she described full of disgust: "I addressed her with the following

---

35 FSAK, Cleve, Letters of the sisters 1845–1854, Sign.: 1337, Dorothee Haube, 21.1.1852.
36 FSAK, Cleve, Letters of the sisters 1845–1854, Sign.: 1337, Dorothee Haube, 21.1.1852.
37 Jansen (2003).
38 FSAK, Cleve, Letters of the sisters 1845–1854, Sign.: 1337, Dorothee Haube, 21.1.1852.
39 FSAK, Cleve, Letters of the sisters 1845–1854, Sign.: 1337, Dorothee Haube, 21.1.1852.

words: Oh Lehna, Lehna – to think of all the things that accompany sin!"[40] In her attempt to allow the sinful patient to die in peace, Sister Dorothee called for a pastor as a last effort, but he had to go home without having achieved anything. Only when the patient could do no longer without the deaconess's help she allowed the nurse to bring some order into her house. From now on, the deaconess in whom this impious dying patient evoked uncanny feelings, visited the dying woman only in the company of another deaconess. In this case the critically ill patient successfully resisted the efforts for spiritual cleanliness. The deaconess admitted this as defeat since she had to take along a second deaconess as support during her visits.

Both case studies document the disciplinary demands which the deaconesses imposed on the poor during their visits. While many deaconesses probably only learned about the bourgeois standards of cleanliness in Kaiserswerth, their "missionary" behavior (in a double sense)[41] prevented them from gaining direct access to the people in the impoverished neighborhoods. They repeatedly met resistance and stubbornness in those whom they wanted to convert to a hygienic conscience and to the Christian faith. Other case stories also illustrate that the community deaconesses and their religiously oriented hygiene efforts met with resistance from those they set out to teach.

Conclusion

For the deaconesses from Kaiserswerth health care included both caring for body and soul and cleaning the house, body and soul. By cleaning their houses and providing poor people with clean and proper clothes, the community deaconesses introduced bourgeois standards of hygiene to the mainly proletarian families. The first cleaning of the living spaces can be compared to a ritual with which the deaconesses not only created outer visible order in the poor quarters but, in a moral and religious sense, also symbolically started to bring order into the patients' lives. After all, the dirt, the disorder and the infestation with vermin was perceived as the outer expression of the desolate soul state of the patients and the poor. At the same time, the deaconesses'

---

40 FSAK, Cleve, Letters of the sisters 1845–1854, Sign.: 1337, Dorothee Haube, 21.1.1852.

41 With his writings on the work of community deaconesses, Fliedner indeed participated in the contemporary colonial discourse. He regarded his deaconesses "as a holy host of native missionaries [...] who brings Christ's mercy to the deserted sick people, neglected children, fallen poor, lost prisoners of a whole country, [...] who, while drying the tears of earthly misery, helps awaken a divine sadness about the misery of sin, but simultaneously helps prevent many earthly and spiritual hardships". Letter from 8th February 1837 by Theodor Fliedner to Amalie Sieveking, persuading her to become principal of the deaconess motherhouse in Kaiserswerth, Staatsarchiv Hamburg, Best. 622-1, Familienarchiv (family archive) Sieveking III, Sign.: I B, Letters to Amalie Sieveking, No. 533, transcribed by Büttner (forthcoming in Hoff (2010)). Furthermore, he compared the life and circumstances of the poor to those of the "savages" on a foreign continent. Cf. Fliedner (1860), p. 77.

cleanliness reflected their striving for inner moral-religious purity. During the first half of the nineteenth century, cleanliness became the central quality of a "good" trained nurse. Not only due to their robes that looked more like bourgeois dresses but also because they represented the bourgeois virtue of "cleanliness", the deaconesses, who mainly came from a rural background, were socially promoted by going to the poor as ambassadors of bourgeois hygiene concepts and practices. They were able not only to distinguish themselves from the proletarian poor people, they also described "cleanliness" as an important means of distinction from the paid untrained careworkers who came from poorer backgrounds. By the beginning of the twentieth century, the concept of personal "cleanliness" had apparently established itself as a nurse's quality and no longer needed to be advertised as a particular requirement. A "sense of cleanliness" was rather seen as part of the female disposition and hence women – by now of all classes – were regarded as more suitable caregivers than men. Now, the future nurses had to be taught the skills of cleanliness in microbiological terms.[42]

Some patients regarded the tidying of the household and the care for the soul as an unauthorized violation of their private sphere. As a consequence they withdrew from the hands of the community deaconesses who were at the time also characterized as the "regulators of all things" in a double meaning. Of course, there are letters from the deaconesses that tell success stories, where families gratefully accepted the cleaning of their house and the efforts of religious purification. The reports of the nurses document the first contact of the protestant missionaries with the social conditions in the impoverished neighborhoods and their first efforts to evoke in the proletarian families an awareness of health similar to that of the religiously awakened middle class.

In conclusion, the letters of community deaconesses allow us to expand the research on bourgeois hygiene efforts, adding the dimension of the history of religion and specifically addressing the everyday practice of piety and faith. Frevert characterized the nurses of the nineteenth century as assistants of the academic physicians who began to establish themselves in the lower classes. However, more recent studies of nineteenth century nursing care revealed that in Christian health care, the tasks of the nurses were regarded as an independent area.[43] For that reason we can conclude that the hygiene attempts of the deaconesses should not only be seen in the context of medical concepts

---

42 See Rupprecht (1908), pp. 17–18. Cf. also Billroth (1881), pp. 6–7, and Rumpf (1900), p. 13: The training for cleanliness is now considered in the context of bacteriology. In order to avoid the transmission and spreading of pathogenic germs, the nurse had to "ensure most thorough cleanliness of all objects". Thus, the idea was here, to teach cleanliness awareness in a microbiological sense. Cf. also Bum (1917), pp. 212–213. The manual by chief staff surgeon Dr. Salzwedel, who worked at the Charité in Berlin and taught at the school for nurses, still emphasizes both "inner" and "outer" cleanliness as important qualities for nurses. However, in addition to a morally impeccable behavior, Salzwedel especially highlights qualities such as "conscientiousness" and "obedience" which were useful for doctors. Salzwedel (1904), pp. XXVIII–XXXI.

43 Cf. Weber-Reich (2003); Nolte (2010); Nolte (2008).

but rather as a central goal of the inner mission that wanted to tackle both the physical-material and spiritual-religious misery of the poor.

Bibliography

Published Sources

Billroth, Theodor: Die Krankenpflege im Hause und im Hospitale. Ein Handbuch für Familien und Krankenpflegerinnen. Wien 1881.

Bum, Anton: Handbuch der Krankenpflege. Berlin 1917.

Disselhoff, Julius: Aus der Diakonissen-Arbeit. In: Der Armen- und Krankenfreund 32 (March/April 1880), pp. 59–76.

Fliedner, Theodor: Das Amt der Gemeinde-Diakonissen. In: Der Armen- und Krankenfreund 12 (March/April 1860), pp. 71–87.

Krügelstein, Franz Christian Karl: Handbuch der allgemeinen Krankenpflege. Zum Gebrauch für Ärzte und Familienväter. Erfurt 1807.

Nightingale, Florence: Notes on nursing: What it is, and what it is not. London 1860.

Rumpf, Theodor: Leidenfaden der Krankenpflege. Leipzig 1900.

Rupprecht, Paul: Die Krankenpflege im Frieden und im Kriege. Leipzig 1908.

Salzwedel, Julius Rudolph Wilhelm: Handbuch der Krankenpflege. Zum Gebrauch für die Krankenwartschule des Kgl. Charité-Krankenhauses sowie zum Selbstunterricht. Berlin 1904.

Selbstprüfungsfragen für Diakonissen und Probeschwestern. In: Der Armen- und Krankenfreund 7 (September/October 1855), pp. 10–17.

Literature

Bashford, Alison: Purity and Pollution. Gender, Embodiment and Victorian Medicine. Basingstoke 1998.

Büttner, Annett: Fliedner-Kulturstiftung in Kaiserswerth. In: Hoff, Walburga (ed.): Religion und Soziale Arbeit. Eine kommentierte Quellensammlung über die Bedeutung von Religion in der Geschichte der Sozialen Arbeit. (= Schriftenreihe des Comenius-Instituts Münster) (forthcoming in 2010).

Douglas, Mary: Purity and Danger: an analysis of concepts of pollution and taboo. London 1966.

Felgentreff, Ruth: Das Diakoniewerk Kaiserswerth 1836–1998. Von der Diakonissenanstalt zum Diakoniewerk – ein Überblick. Düsseldorf 1998.

Frevert, Ute: The Civilizing Tendency of Hygiene. Working-Class Women under Medical Control in Imperial Germany. In: Fout, John C. (ed.): German Women in the Nineteenth Century. A Social History. London 1984, pp. 320–345.

Frevert, Ute: "Fürsorgliche Belagerung." Hygienebewegung und Arbeiterfrauen im 19. und 20. Jahrhundert. In: Geschichte und Gesellschaft 11 (1985), pp. 420–446.

Hoff, Walburga (ed.): Religion und Soziale Arbeit. Eine kommentierte Quellensammlung über die Bedeutung von Religion in der Geschichte der Sozialen Arbeit. (= Schriftenreihe des Comenius-Instituts Münster) (forthcoming in 2010).

Jansen, Sarah: "Schädlinge." Geschichte eines wissenschaftlichen und politischen Konstrukts 1840–1920. Frankfurt/Main; New York 2003.

Klein, Walter: "Sie sehen mir alle freundlichen Gesichtes entgegen." Die Beziehung zwischen Patienten und Krankenschwestern im Saarbrücker Bürgerhospital in der Mitte des 19. Jahrhunderts. In: Medizin, Gesellschaft und Geschichte 21 (2002), pp. 93–120.

Köser, Silke: Denn eine Diakonisse darf kein Alltagsmensch sein. Kollektive Identitäten Kaiserswerther Diakonissen 1836–1914. Leipzig 2006.

Kreutzer, Susanne: Vom "Liebesdienst" zum modernen Frauenberuf. Die Reform der Krankenpflege nach 1945. Frankfurt/Main; New York 2005.

Labisch, Alfons: Homo hygienicus. Gesundheit und Medizin in der Neuzeit. Frankfurt/Main; New York 1992.

Löneke, Regina; Spieker, Ira (eds.): Reinliche Leiber – Schmutzige Geschäfte. Körperhygiene und Reinlichkeitsvorstellungen in zwei Jahrhunderten. Göttingen 1996.

Nolte, Karen: Telling the painful truth – Nurses and physicians in the nineteenth century. In: Nursing History Review 16 (2008), pp. 115–134.

Nolte, Karen: Pflege von Sterbenden im 19. Jahrhundert – eine ethikgeschichtliche Annäherung. In: Kreutzer, Susanne (ed.): Transformationen pflegerischen Handelns. Institutionelle Kontexte und soziale Praxis vom 19. zum 21. Jahrhundert. Osnabrück 2010, pp. 87–108.

Sarasin, Philipp: Reizbare Maschinen. Eine Geschichte des Körpers 1765–1914. Frankfurt/Main 2001.

Schmidt, Jutta: Beruf: Schwester. Mutterhausdiakonie im 19. Jahrhundert. Frankfurt/Main; New York 1998.

Seidler, Eduard; Leven, Karl-Heinz: Geschichte der Medizin und der Krankenpflege. Stuttgart 2003.

Weber-Reich, Traudel: "Wir sind die Pionierinnen der Pflege …". Krankenschwestern und ihre Pflegestätten im 19. Jahrhundert am Beispiel Göttingens. Bern 2003.

The rise and fall of the *Fürsorgerin* (female welfare worker) in Austrian public health policies.
Theory and practice of a professional link within a changing social and epidemiological framework

Andreas Weigl

The lack of a professional link in social and health policy

From the turn of the century to the years leading up to World War I the main issues of sanitary reform shifted from hardware – sewers and water supply, to software – individual people. In particular the quality of mothering and infant care became central issues of social policy.[1] On the basis of achievements in the new scientific field of bacteriology, far-reaching improvements in public health seemed possible and the mortality dropped to a rate that not even experts would have thought possible one or two generations earlier. But the reformers did not only come from among the medical profession and the sanitary movement. The idea of a healthy people's body ("Volkskörper") was spread widely by a variety of professions such as economists, military planners, social politicians, philanthropists and the women's lib movement. Many of them shared the idea of a preventive social medicine that came close to eugenic and humane economic attitudes.[2]

The demographic circumstances obviously stimulated optimistic hopes. Infant mortality rates decreased sharply everywhere in Europe with the Habsburg Monarchy being no exception. Nevertheless the level of infant mortality was still high. Even in the years before the outbreak of war, 20% of all newborns died within their first year of life. In the Alpine lands, the later Republic of Austria, the figure was 18%.[3] Although there was no doubt that infant and child care improvements were of major importance for the future of the Monarchy, sanitary reform was hampered by the anachronistic structures of the poor relief institutions that were in place. The expertises and records of the first Congress of Child Welfare in Vienna in 1907 clearly reflect this problem. As in Germany, a lot of the measures planned and taken by public authorities focused exclusively on children born out of wedlock, foster children and children in institutional care. The living conditions of these children were observed by wealthy volunteers from the upper and middle classes who had no professional knowledge of medicine or sanitation and whose mindset was

---

1 Rollet (1997), p. 42; Porter (1999), p. 174; Fildes (1992).
2 For the Austrian discussion see Baader/Hofer/Mayer (2007), pp. 31–207; Melinz/Zimmermann (1991), p. 162.
3 Chesnais (1992), p. 63; Vallin (1991), pp. 50–52; Pirquet (1927); Statistik Austria (2007), p. 215.

separated from that of the needy by a wide class gap.[4] As Ilse Arlt, one of the eminent Austrian reformers, noted: "Over the previous 25 years the high infant mortality had become an important issue of medical science and paediatrics and infant care finally developed quite well. Yet both neglected to deal with the care of children after infancy and therefore a lot of infants who had survived their first year of life died later due to poor care."[5]

One of the main issues of social reform was therefore the creation of a new job profile for professionally trained welfare workers. This professional link was to guarantee a much higher degree of "medicalization" of working class mothers than breastfeeding-propaganda or similar activities could achieve. Three reformers were of major importance in the process of defining, creating and establishing this new profession in Austria: Ilse Arlt, Julius Tandler and Leopold Moll.

Reformers: Moll, Arlt and Tandler

After the turn of the century the conditions for reform were most favourable in the field of infant and child care. In 1908 the "Für das Kind!"-campaign of Emperor Franz Joseph I called for donations to establish the Emperor's Jubilee Fund that would sponsor orphanages, clinics and children's programs all over the Habsburg Empire. A Centre for Child Protection and Youth Welfare was founded as an umbrella group for regional youth welfare branches.[6] In 1910 it was decided that the fund would finance the construction and management of the "Reichsanstalt für Mütter- und Säuglingsfürsorge", a multifunctional institution that included a paediatric hospital and a school for child care. Leopold Moll, a Prague born paediatrician[7], became head of planning management and later of the institution itself. What was most innovative about his project was that the school would offer its graduates a combined qualification as infant welfare workers as well as hospital nurses. Moll argued that many of the female students of this school would not be aware of their vocational aptitude as far as these two closely related professions were concerned. The secondary goal of this combined training was to give the new profession of infant welfare worker a solid medical grounding. The duties of the infant welfare workers included working in mothers' consultation clinics under the guidance of the paediatricians and making home visits. Although their qualification was similar to that of nurses, their field of activity differed geographically. In Moll's concept, these welfare workers were mainly to work in the field, especially in small towns and rural areas.[8] Actually, the first professional infant welfare workers – initially only intended for children taken care of by the city, later for

---

4   Erster Österreichischer Kinderschutzkongress (1907); Stöckel (1996), pp. 196–238.
5   Arlt (1921), p. 126.
6   Healy (2004), p. 217.
7   Lesky (1981), p. 195; Moll (1919), pp. 5–9.
8   Moll (1919), pp. 56–69.

all illegitimate children – were employed by the city of Vienna in 1914. Their number rose from 6 in 1914 to 13 in 1915 and eventually 18 in 1916[9], obviously much too small a number to substantially improve the situation of infants. There were some similarities with the training of tuberculosis welfare workers, a profession that emerged during World War I. But these welfare workers required only a nurse's training and some additional 2-year courses.[10]

The concept of a new female profession, the *Fürsorgerin* (female welfare worker) on a broader scale – as a professional link between physicians and those in need of care – was not originally Moll's idea. Among the forerunners were British Health Visitors in Welfare Centres[11], some female infant welfare workers employed at a maternity clinic in Paris since 1892[12] and the "Recherche-Schwestern" at the "Säuglingsfürsorgestellen" (infant welfare and mothers' consultation clinics) introduced in Berlin and Munich and, from 1905, in other German cities[13]. Indeed the concept had not been proposed by a member of the medical profession but by Ilse Arlt[14] at the "Congress of public poor relief" in Copenhagen in 1910[15]. Although Arlt's father, an oculist, grew up in an upper middle class family with a strong connection to academic medicine, it was poverty that became her favourite field of interest. With support from the Viennese economist and social scientist Eugen von Philippovich, she was allowed to take part in lectures in economics, medicine and pedagogy at Vienna University for two years. It was, however, not possible for Arlt to take a normal degree in economics. At the time, female students were not admitted to the faculty of law. Nevertheless, it was economics and not medicine that interested her most.[16] In this respect her biography shows similarities with that of Alice Salomon in Berlin, who had also studied economics. In general, economics became very important for the "science" of public care.[17]

Initially Arlt's approach to a reform in public relief based on professional care was close to that of physicians such as Moll. For Arlt, as she wrote some years later, public relief was educational in the eighteenth century, economical and judicial in the nineteenth and now, in the twentieth century, it was medical.[18] But she applied the term "medical" in a sense that differed from the concepts of many male medical reformers. Arlt's ultimate goal was to establish a genuinely new profession beyond the mere assistance to physicians and bureaucrats, a profession focused on what could be called Arlt's version of "social case work". In 1912 Arlt, like her contemporary Alice Salomon in Berlin,

9   Mittermeier (1994), pp. 109–110.
10 Dietrich-Daum (2007), p. 258.
11 Fehlemann/Vögele (2002), pp. 42–43.
12 Köstler (1930), p. 282.
13 Sachße (2003), pp. 62–65.
14 For a biographical sketch see Simon (2002).
15 Steinhauser (1994), p. 112.
16 Frey (2005), pp. 27–31.
17 Frey (2005), pp. 55–69, 100–101; Sachße (2003), p. 87.
18 Arlt (1921), p. 80.

founded a private school in Vienna called "Vereinigte Fachkurse für Volks-
pflege" (combined courses in public relief). This was one of the first, maybe
even the first, school worldwide that offered a general and professional education for welfare workers, although similar schools existed in Berlin, Cologne
and Heidelberg.[19] In Arlt's school the students not only received basic training
in poor relief and child care, like in Salomon's school in Berlin they were also
taught what Arlt referred to as "care science", a social science that examined
the reasons for poverty as well as the living standards of the poor.[20] Although
this science did not officially exist at the time, there was no lack of studies
dealing with poverty from a different angle.

Soon after the outbreak of war in 1914, the demand for welfare workers
rose dramatically and Arlt's school became the prototype for several others
that were founded during World War I and afterwards: e. g. in Vienna in 1916,
Lower Austria in 1922, Upper Austria in 1926 and Styria in 1915.[21] Many of
them specialized in youth and family care, Moll's school in infant care. It was
only Arlt's school that offered a full training in public care.

Now it was up to the public sector to create jobs for professional welfare
workers besides the small number of infant welfare workers. In 1916 a Youth
Welfare Office was founded in Vienna and in 1917 the "Academy of Social
Administration" of the City of Vienna was opened.[22] Other cities followed.
The Youth Welfare Office of the City of Linz opened in 1917.[23] The "Academy" in Vienna, although in fact only a centre offering courses for *Fürsorgerinnen*[24], became the most important of its kind during the interwar period. The
man behind the extension of these activities to a much broader scale was Julius Tandler (1869–1936). Tandler, the son of a poor Moravian Jewish family,
was born in Iglau (Jihlava). In the 1870s the family went to Vienna, where he
studied medicine and became a distinguished anatomist at Vienna University.[25] In 1917 Tandler convinced Emperor Karl I to establish a ministry of public care ("Ministerium für soziale Fürsorge") and later a ministry of public
health. This step led to state regulation of the formerly private sector of poor
relief.[26]

Tandler, who became undersecretary for public health in the post-war
government[27], failed to introduce a powerful public care policy at the level of
the central state, the new Republic of Austria, just like contemporary reformers in Weimar Germany[28]. The "Kommunalhygiene" (Adolf Gottstein), the

19 Steinhauser (1994), p. 112; Frey (2005), p. 41.
20 Ertl (1995), p. 35; Frey (2005), pp. 42–43.
21 Steinhauser (1994), pp. 110–111.
22 Mittermeier (1994), pp. 112–114.
23 Kepplinger (2001), p. 727.
24 Simon (1993), p. 15.
25 Sablik (1983), pp. 11, 21–84.
26 Sablik (1983), pp. 140–141; Steinhauser (1994), pp. 27, 32–33.
27 Sablik (1983), pp. 159–160.
28 Stöckel (1996), p. 306.

communication of the socio-hygienic principles inherent in sanitary reform to the target groups at the municipal level, remained the driving force of sanitary reform.[29] After the collapse of the post-war coalition of Social Democrats and Christian Social party in the summer of 1920, Tandler switched to the Vienna city administration and became the city's councillor of welfare. In this political function he proceeded to alter the vision and practice of public health and social welfare and started an ambitious welfare program. Child care became one of its main issues. On the one hand, Tandler stated that society was committed to assist every child in need, on the other hand, he made it a condition for receiving public support that parents took care of their children as was to be expected of "respectable" families.[30] No doubt Tandler's conception of welfare policies was not only that of preventive medicine, but to some extent eugenic too.[31] In practice this led to a shift in welfare budgets from poor relief – focused on elderly people – to infant, child and youth care.[32]

The establishment of *Fürsorgerinnen* in community services

Tandler knew that he required somebody who was in contact with the working class to implement his idea of a general public welfare policy for the whole Viennese population. Therefore, the number of *Fürsorgerinnen* – an occupational term officially created by the City Council of Vienna in April 1917 – was raised rapidly from 91 in 1918 to 278 in 1931.[33]

Although Tandler stressed the role of the *Fürsorgerinnen* in his concept of public care and welfare policy, he, like many other male physicians and bureaucrats[34], set lower standards for their qualifications than Arlt because for him they were mainly assistants to the medical staff[35]. Later he became interested in psychology and enabled female members of the Psychological Institute of the University of Vienna to conduct tests with children in the "Kinderübernahmestelle". This was a children's diagnostic service for those who were taken away from their parents if the municipality judged them to be deficient in nurturing capability and responsibility.[36] This process was initiated by *Fürsorgerinnen* on the grounds of their experiences in homes, schools and orphanages.[37]

29   Gottstein (1975), p. 237.
30   Melinz/Zimmermann (1994), p. 288.
31   Jancsy (1982), pp. 123–126.
32   Melinz/Unger (1996), p. 31.
33   Mittermeier (1994), pp. 112–113; Gemeinde Wien (1933), p. 30.
34   For the German discourse see Stöckel (2002), p. 59.
35   Ziering (2002), p. 20.
36   Gruber (1991), pp. 68, 71.
37   Wolfgruber (1997), pp. 79–100.

In contrast to the old poor relief system of the nineteenth century that had
a vast majority of male visitors[38], the female conception of the profession was
undisputed. "Tandler and most leading socialists believed that a special 'female empathy' was necessary for the often emotional demands on welfare
workers."[39] In a textbook for public care visitors published in 1930 Viktor
Gegenbauer, the head of the city's health office, characterized social hygiene
as the "child" of a rational, scientific father (medicine) and a careful mother
(the female welfare workers).[40] On the level of public discourse, the children
and youth welfare system in Red Vienna was embedded within the construction of the idea of a public motherhood, of the city administration as a supra-
mother of all of its children.[41] Indicative of this, a fountain sculpture created
by the sculptor Anton Hanak for the garden of the "Kinderübernahmestelle",
which can be found today in the city hall park in the Wien-Mauer quarter in
the 23rd district of Vienna, bears the title "caring mother".[42]

However, outside of Vienna the dominant image of the *Fürsorgerinnen* profession was very close to that of a nun. There, *Fürsorgerinnen* often wore a
Catholic nun's habit and were addressed as "sister".[43]

The Viennese public welfare system as introduced in Red Vienna in the
early twenties was not at all unique. It showed many similarities with systems
in German cities such as Düsseldorf.[44] But its general approach went further
than many contemporary activities of other communities. Most of the *Fürsorgerinnen* in Red Vienna and in Austria were mainly a kind of general youth
welfare worker, comparable to the "Wohlfahrtspflegerinnen" (female welfare
worker) in Weimar Germany, but not as specialized as tuberculosis health visitors such as the "infirmière visiteuse" in France and "Gesundheitsfürsorgerin-
nen" in Germany.[45] In the mid twenties about 45% of home visits by *Fürsorgerinnen* were to school children.[46] They visited poor families of the visitor
districts on a regular basis and checked their living conditions, mainly the
child care of unmarried mothers and foster families.[47] The same process took
place with regard to all newborn children from municipal hospitals, where
infant welfare workers registered all babies born in hospitals as well as all
home births[48], a procedure that was established in many English cities before
World War I[49]. Most newborn children were visited only once or at the most

---

38 Mittermeier (1994), p. 103.
39 Gruber (1991), p. 70; Kepplinger (2001), p. 735.
40 Gegenbauer (1930), pp. 12–13.
41 Wolfgruber (1999), p. 292.
42 Vienna Municipal and Provincial Archives (Wiener Stadt- und Landesarchiv), Foto-
    sammlung Gerlach C 18604M. See Weihsmann (1985), p. 292.
43 Kepplinger (2001), p. 735.
44 Gruber (1991), p. 66.
45 Geiger (2006), p. 180; Rosenhaupt (1927); Köstler (1930), p. 288.
46 Gemeinde Wien (1927), p. 396.
47 Mittermeier (1994), pp. 116–117.
48 Gemeinde Wien (1927), p. 380.
49 Fehlemann/Vögele (2002), p. 44.

occasionally. As Julius Tandler stressed: "It is the task of the *Fürsorgerin* to visit every mother. If conditions are good, this first visit is naturally also the last."[50] For the middle and upper classes the most annoying innovation was the distribution of infant layettes to all newborns as a "birthday present" from the municipality. This activity, which was to an extent a "Trojan horse" approach, began in 1927. It gave welfare workers the chance to check the home of every parent, even in the case of rich people.[51] But this was only a side effect. The main goal of the visits to working class families was the education of the mothers in the "mothering profession".[52] The number of visits increased steadily: e. g. in 1922 welfare workers carried out 189,000 and in 1925 213,000 visits, a level that remained stable in the following years.[53] Besides these visits, the so-called "Verbindungsdienste" (linkage activities) in primary schools, maternity clinics and kindergartens were another source of information. And it was this part of their job that brought them into contact with the medical staff in the public health sector, especially paediatricians in schools and gynaecologists.[54] In many cases they really only served as assistants, for instance measuring the temperature or weight of the babies.[55] A joint visit to the doctor and *Fürsorgerin* was scheduled for all foster children in public or private care and for all illegitimately born children.[56] Besides their work in mothers' consultation clinics, it were above all criminal law cases of child abuse or murder which led to the *Fürsorgerinnen* having to involve doctors.[57]

The training of public welfare workers in medical subjects was quite thorough. Health care, infant care, social hygiene and basic knowledge in anamnesis were taught next to practical work in institutions of public care.[58] As one of the early students in Ilse Arlt's school, Rosa Dworschak, remembered, a certain degree of medical knowledge was absolutely necessary to pass the exams.[59] From 1930, textbooks like those of the Academy of Social Administration of the City of Vienna included chapters on health statistics, dietetics and social medicine, especially aetiology of infectious diseases.[60] Some of the *Fürsorgerinnen* complained about a certain over-emphasis on theory.[61] The high qualification standards that required six years of attending a grammar school ("Gymnasium") – or a similar secondary school – and a minimum age of 20 meant that almost 100% of girls in this profession came from the upper or at

---

50 Tandler (1925), p. 8.
51 Pirhofer/Sieder (1982), p. 332; Gruber (1991), p. 69.
52 Wolfgruber (1999), p. 292.
53 Gemeinde Wien (1927), p. 396; Gemeinde Wien (1933), p. 30.
54 Mittermeier (1994), p. 116.
55 Lichtenberg (1932), p. 38; Dietrich-Daum (2007), p. 259.
56 Melinz/Zimmermann (1994), p. 299.
57 Smekal-Huber (1936), p. 3.
58 Steinhauser (1994), pp. 112–113, 219–225.
59 Steinhauser (1994), p. 117.
60 Gemeinde Wien (1930).
61 Köstler (1930), p. 293.

least middle classes.[62] Especially daughters of high ranking civil servants were overrepresented.[63] In 1930, 58% of the public welfare workers had "Matura" (A-levels) and 8% were university graduates.[64] Given the high proportion of Jewish girls among better educated women[65], it is probable that some of the *Fürsorgerinnen* came from the enlightened, bourgeois community of assimilated Jews who sympathized with the Social Democrat movement. However, a majority of Jewish women, even those who were active in the liberal-bourgeois women's movement, became increasingly involved in private Jewish associations as Jewish people in need were habitually confronted with anti-Semitism and reproached for a lack of willingness to integrate by the authorities, which increased the need for Jewish welfare organizations.[66] In 1930 the welfare activities of these organizations were centralized in the "Fürsorgezentrale der Israelitischen Kultusgemeinde" (General welfare office of the Viennese Jewish Community).[67] The records of the candidates for municipal welfare workers indicate that there was a clear predominance of candidates from a Catholic background and this is confirmed by biographical historical accounts.[68] This was even more true outside of Vienna. In Linz, for instance, an extensive continuity of *Fürsorgerinnen* personnel can be established for the time period 1920–1945.[69]

However, in the mid 1920s remarkable changes occurred. The curriculum was modified. Medical subjects became less important, psychology and practical "social work" became the main subjects.[70] As in Germany, the profession became more and more a job in public services like any other, and no longer a "vocation".[71] Because of the culture gap between bourgeois welfare workers and their mainly working class clients, steps to open the profession to working class girls were introduced. In 1926 the job of assistant welfare worker was introduced in Vienna, with much lower educational requirements.[72] This category of *Fürsorgerinnen* nonetheless remained very much in the minority. In the year 1931 for instance there were 204 (primary) *Hauptfürsorgerinnen* and only 74 (assistant) *Hilfsfürsorgerinnen*[73], not least because the hiring and equali-

---

62 Mittermeier (1994), pp. 113–114; Wolfgruber (1997), p. 63.
63 Ziering (2002), p. 20.
64 Mittermeier (1994), p. 116.
65 Rozenblit (1983), pp. 118–122.
66 Malleier (2006), p. 263; Hecht (2008), p. 53.
67 Malleier (2003), p. 109.
68 Vienna Municipal and Provincial Archives (Wiener Stadt- und Landesarchiv), Municipal Department 207 A 26 5–8; Autobiographical Interview of Reinhard Sieder with Mrs. Oče, born 1901, *Fürsorgerin* of the City of Vienna in 1927–1938.
69 Kepplinger (2001), p. 736.
70 Steinhauser (1994), p. 44; Wolfgruber (1997), pp. 69–70.
71 Sachße (2003), pp. 215, 224.
72 Mittermeier (1994), pp. 114–115.
73 Gemeinde Wien (1933), p. 30.

zation of the assistant *Fürsorgerinnen* met with embittered resistance from the (primary) *Fürsorgerinnen*[74].

As far as the role of welfare workers in public health is concerned there was a wide regional gap between Vienna and the rest of the country during the interwar period. In Vienna the welfare workers were to some extent metamorphosed into public health nurses.[75] In the provinces of Austria, the legal framework of the old poor relief system remained more or less unchanged.[76] Parts of the Viennese model were adopted nonetheless and the number of *Fürsorgerinnen* at the federal state and local authority level rose rapidly.[77] In 1934, 1,439 *Fürsorgerinnen* were employed in public and private institutions all over Austria, 631 of these in Vienna.[78] The wide gap between Vienna and the rest of the country can be observed in the activities of tuberculosis health visitors. In 1934, 36% of patients in tuberculosis care centres in Vienna were admitted by welfare workers, in the public care districts of Linz and Salzburg only 6–7%.[79]

Since the early 1930s, a decrease in the importance of the link between the medical profession and the *Fürsorgerinnen* can be observed. The reasons for the changing job profile of welfare workers were both demographical and economical. In terms of welfare policy, the heavy decrease in infant and child mortality and in tuberculosis mortality as well as the increased hospitalization of birth[80] diminished the role of health visiting compared to other fields of social policy. In the interwar period infant mortality in Austria decreased from 16% to 9%, tuberculosis mortality shrank to one third of its 1919 level.[81] Economically, the consequences of the Great Depression forced the Social Democrats and later on the Christian Social regime to shift their budget back to the more traditional fields of poor relief, which concerned unemployment and the elderly.[82] The overall trend towards an increased emphasis on the role of psychology in the job profile of the *Fürsorgerinnen* continued throughout the years of the Austro-Clerical dictatorship though its ideological justification shifted from Marxism to Catholicism.[83]

After the "Anschluss" in March 1938, which brought the Nazis to power, the trend was totally reversed. In Nazi ideology traditional poor relief and welfare policy were regarded as counterproductive. The main goal of social

---

74 Vienna Municipal and Provincial Archives (Wiener Stadt- und Landesarchiv), Municipal Department 207 A 28 3, Draft of a letter of the employee representation of the municipal *Fürsorgerinnen* to the "Association of white-collar employees of the City of Vienna" (Verband der Angestellten der Stadt Wien), Vienna, 10.3.1929.
75 Simon (1982), p. 114.
76 For Upper Austria see Kepplinger (2001), pp. 715–797, 719.
77 Kepplinger (2001), pp. 729, 735.
78 Bundesamt für Statistik (1935), p. 310.
79 Dietrich-Daum (2007), p. 281.
80 Weigl (2000), pp. 211, 244.
81 Kytir (1989), p. 54; Dietrich-Daum (2007), p. 265.
82 Melinz/Unger (1996), pp. 46–50.
83 Melinz/Zimmermann (1994), pp. 289, 301.

policy was to "enhance the status of the inherently healthy population".[84] Therefore, the role of the welfare workers, now called *Volkspflegerinnen* (people's welfare workers) was on the one hand to support "healthy Arians", especially by encouraging mothers to bear as many children as possible, on the other hand to control the unfit, the disabled and to some extent support euthanasia. In 1943 Kamilla Heidenreich, head of the "Soziale Frauenschule", the successor school to the Academy of Social Administration, described the job of a *Volkspflegerin* in terms of Nazi-ideology: "the job of the *Volkspflegerin* is [...] one of the most important in people's welfare and people's health, because she eliminates the incurable from the vigorous and average of the people's community."[85]

This led to radical changes concerning the admission to the job. From now on membership in the NSDAP, the Nazi-party, was required in addition to knowledge and practical experience, especially in the field of infant care. Other qualifications, especially graduation from secondary education ("Matura"), were no longer of any importance. Training in the "Soziale Frauenschule" now included the subject "Genetic imprinting and racial care" as well as an increase in practical work experience in hospitals and similar institutions.[86]

The attitude of the Nazi rulers towards the importance of the *Volkspflegerinnen* was contradictory. On the one hand, they were needed to implement Nazi racial policy in families and homes, on the other hand, in Nazi-"survival of the fittest"-ideology Arians did not really need support on account of their superiority.[87] This conflict was reflected in the growing appointments of *Volkspflegerinnen* for secretarial and administrative work during the war in the genetic imprinting database ("erbbiologische Bestandsaufnahme") which took place alongside an increased need for welfare work in orphanages and military hospitals.[88]

Nevertheless, the demand for *Volkspflegerinnen* still increased, corresponding to the totalitarian approach of the regime. There was, however, a lack of students. Education costs were quite high compared to those of primary school teachers for instance, the jobs were badly paid and the alternatives for well-educated (upper) middle class girls on the labour market as well as – thinking in terms of Nazi population policy – the "marriage market" were much more attractive.[89]

---

84 Sachße/Tennstedt (1992), p. 250.
85 Geiger (2006), p. 183.
86 Geiger (2006), pp. 181–184.
87 Steinhauser (1994), p. 53.
88 Geiger (2006), p. 184; Czech (2007).
89 Sachße/Tennstedt (1992), pp. 196–197; Geiger (2006), pp. 178–179.

(Medical) Practices

Diaries and reports of female welfare workers from the 1920s and 1930s mirror an emphasis on psychological work and the traditional poor-relief activities of the *Fürsorgerinnen*.[90] The main link to medical issues was their monitoring function. They were present when doctors in mothers' consultation clinics ("Mutterberatungen") advised new mothers on child nutrition and childcare. In the case of nutritional problems "nursing samples" were taken: the babies were weighed before and after nursing in the mothers' consultation clinics and if they had gained too little, the reasons for this were investigated. During home visits it was their task to check whether mothers were putting the doctor's advice into practice.[91] The same procedure was carried out alongside paediatricians in schools. Other activities were limited to simple assistance in mothers' consultation clinics.[92] In cases where child abuse and homicide of children had to be testified, it was the duty of the *Fürsorgerinnen* to consult physicians.[93] But in general, as the evidence of oral history shows, their approach to medicalization was focused on clean, tidy houses and the running of "proper" homes.[94]

Nevertheless, in some cases this focus on "proper" homes could acquire a medical aspect as two examples illustrate. The first case was reported in a radio speech of 1932 by *Fürsorgerin* Elfriede Lichtenberg:

> In the same house, two floors up, I have a family whose two children had to be taken away two years ago, they are in local authority care and from time to time I go and see if the family's circumstances have improved enough for the children to be sent back. As soon as I come in a terrible smell hits me. The beds are stuffed with rags and have not been aired although it is already midday. Of course there is vermin. In this case nothing can be done, although the mother carried on terribly when the children were taken away and she is attached to them [...].[95]

During the first home visits of the assistant welfare worker Mrs. Oče in 1928, when she accompanied a *Hauptfürsorgerin*, a similar problem occurred:

> And then I had my first experience of an angry mother throwing a burning petrol lamp at me because we took her child away, an absolutely filthy child [...] Before we dared to take the child on the tram we had to wash it in the Youth Welfare Office, it was necessary to use oil to get the dirt off.[96]

Sometimes the *Fürsorgerinnen* also used conflict within the families they visited to obtain information or to find the reasons for aberrant, abnormal behaviour

---

90 Smekal-Huber (1936); Lichtenberg (1932).
91 Pirhofer/Sieder (1982), p. 332; Autobiographical Interview of Reinhard Sieder with Mrs. Oče, born 1901, *Fürsorgerin* of the City of Vienna in 1927–1938.
92 Lichtenberg (1932), p. 38.
93 Wolfgruber (1997), p. 69; Smekal-Huber (1936), p. 3.
94 Pirhofer/Sieder (1982), pp. 333–334.
95 Lichtenberg (1932), p. 37.
96 Autobiographical Interview of Reinhard Sieder with Mrs. Oče, born 1901, *Fürsorgerin* of the City of Vienna in 1927–1938.

of children, like in the following example of a girl who behaved conspicuously at school:

> And chance came to my aid. When a fight breaks out in the family this is always very helpful for the welfare officers because then they all tell on each other. Like at school or among criminals when they grass on someone. An adult came to the Youth Welfare Office and said that the girl was being mistreated by her stepmother. So I went into the house and confronted them there with the allegation that the child was being mistreated by her stepmother. The stepmother went hysterical and screamed blue murder and [...] all the other members of the family tried to calm her down, only my little girl stood in the corner, as if turned to stone, hard and impassive and I took that as my cue. I said since everyone got so upset the child couldn't be normal and took her with me straight away, because when there is a suspicion of mistreatment the youth welfare [...] takes the child away immediately, the only requirement being that an application for an order to remove the child be made to the Children's Court within 8 days; and this has to have a very solid grounding. So I took the risk. [...] And it turned out that the mistreatment consisted in the stepmother lifting the child up and knocking her down. [...] She used to do it again and again.[97]

Since the very beginning and not only in Red Vienna, *Fürsorgerinnen* played a crucial role in an Austrian welfare system based on control coming from a coercive background. This was one of the main differences to the more or less voluntary British system.[98] The disciplinary power was not only in the hands of an anonymous administrative body. Every *Fürsorgerin* exercised individual power too[99]; e. g. in some cases *Fürsorgerinnen* treated infants even worse than the children's own mothers did. One witness remembered that his mother told the *Fürsorgerin* about all his "sins" after which he was beaten regularly by the *Fürsorgerin*.[100] Because this case happened in the Nazi-period it is not a good example for generalization. Other *Fürsorgerinnen* stressed in interviews that they never did any harm to children.[101] But it is no surprise that the acceptance of the *Fürsorgerinnen* was low, because they put heavy pressure on poor families, especially the mothers.[102]

Complaints about the behaviour of welfare workers, about their treatment of the needy, their arrogance in dealing with sick persons needing medical referrals and pharmaceutical prescriptions, as well as their tendency to treat the entire working class like children, were quite common.[103] As long as these complaints were limited to the needy and related to non-violent coercion the image problem was not too bad. But after the "Anschluss" the control system was theoretically extended to include the whole population and the means of coercion became unlimited. Especially the support of what could be called

97 Autobiographical Interview of Reinhard Sieder with Mrs. Oče, born 1901, *Fürsorgerin* of the City of Vienna in 1927–1938.
98 Davies (1988), p. 58.
99 Kepplinger (2001), pp. 730–731.
100 Ziering (2002), p. 27.
101 Autobiographical Interview of Reinhard Sieder with Mrs. Oče, born 1901, *Fürsorgerin* of the City of Vienna in 1927–1938.
102 Pirhofer/Sieder (1982), p. 333.
103 Gruber (1991), p. 71.

"medicine in the service of racial policy" became crucial. Denunciation by a *Volkspflegerin* could lead to death, either in a concentration camp or in clinics specialized in euthanasia. It was also the duty of a *Volkspflegerin* to bring denunciations by other people to the notice of the Nazi authorities.[104] It comes as no surprise that home visits by the *Volkspflegerinnen* were in most cases less than welcome. However, home visits in an atmosphere of fear and animosity were not only characteristic for the Nazi period. A few years before the "Anschluss" a middle class *Fürsorgerin* wrote into her diary:

> I shout, because the door is closed. No answer [...] I shout again, no answer. Just as I am going to ask the neighbours, the window opens. "Who's there?" "The *Fürsorgerin*", I reply and think: Now it is all over, now the people with their guilty conscience won't open the door for me for sure.[105]

Other problems arose because of the class gap between the welfare workers and the needy. For some of the unmarried middle class welfare workers the job was pure economic necessity, the only chance to sustain class-related standards of living[106], but not their favourite way of life at all[107]. Even the highly motivated girls were parted by a wide class gap from the "unrespectable" working class families they visited. During these home visits not only public but also private attitudes of "respectability" clashed with one another.

Even *Hilfsfürsorgerinnen*, who had actually been recruited in order to ameliorate the "cultural clash", often took on the same kinds of behaviour as their bourgeois colleagues. Their inclusion did not after all create any real "closeness" between the *Fürsorgerinnen* and those whose welfare they looked after.[108]

The problem of the "cultural clash" was by no means confined to the big city. Contemporary accounts show the mood in the country was especially critical. Cases are documented in which *Fürsorgerinnen* were terrorized by village youths caterwauling and they were physically threatened.[109] The relationship between the *Fürsorgerinnen* and the older local midwives was also difficult; the midwives often had little knowledge of hygiene and did not want to abandon their traditional midwifery practices.[110]

But the threat of physical violence was just one of several strategies against the welfare workers. Another strategy was to attempt to have decisions made by *Fürsorgerinnen* revoked by their supervisors. One such case is documented in a disciplinary file in the Viennese Youth Welfare Office dating from the year 1932. According to this a Ms P. tried several times to recover her three children who were in public care. She failed to obtain the approval of the *Fürsor-*

---

104 Geiger (2006), pp. 188–189.

105 Smekal-Huber (1936), p. 23.

106 Wolfgruber (1997), p. 63; Frey (2005), p. 50; for Germany see Sachße (2003), pp. 253–254.

107 Smekal-Huber (1936), p. 4.

108 Autobiographical Interview of Reinhard Sieder with Mrs. Oče, born 1901, *Fürsorgerin* of the City of Vienna in 1927–1938.

109 Köstler (1930), pp. 284–285.

110 Report of *Fürsorgerin* Hermine Jakobartl (1925).

gerin Marie P. Ms P. then turned to the supervisor of the *Fürsorgerin*, Magistrats-Sekretär Dr. L., alleging that the *Fürsorgerin* was "rude" to her. According to the records she actually succeeded in persuading Dr. L. that a "transfer" was justified. This decision led to an outburst of anger on the part of the *Fürsorgerin* towards Dr. L. that ended with a disciplinary procedure against the *Fürsorgerin*.[111]

A long term problem arose from the downgrading of educational standards required during the Nazi-period. The downgrading slowly destroyed the welfare workers' professional identity as part of a white-collar female labour market.[112] This became a crucial point in the post-war history of the *Fürsorgerinnen*.

From *Fürsorgerinnen* to social workers

At the end of the war, especially in Vienna, the public authorities tried to re-establish the old organization scheme of Red Vienna. Obviously welfare workers were needed in many fields of public care, due to malnutrition, a short term increase in tuberculosis and a higher mortality rate due to other infectious diseases and a lack of almost all means. But after a few years it became quite clear that the image of the profession was damaged and continuously declining. The lowering of required educational standards continued. This further increased the distance between the *Fürsorgerin* profession and the public health sector. A survey on the reputation of female professions by the opinion research institute IFES in the 1960s showed the *Fürsorgerinnen* ranking last but one in female jobs, only slightly above chemical cleaners.[113]

In the 1960s and 1970s the concern of public care shifted from material poverty to psychosocial problems. In 1963 educational standards were upgraded once again and taught in the "Lehranstalten für gehobene Sozialberufe" (schools for higher ranking social professions). In general the "Matura" (A-levels) was required and the curriculum included far more elements of "social work", which meant less medicine and more psychology than previously.[114] But it took until the late 1970s for the old-fashioned *Fürsorgerin* job profile to be totally refashioned into that of modern social workers with an emphasis on social casework with methodological competence, as had been called for so long ago by reformers such as Ilse Arlt and Mary Richmond.[115]

---

111 Vienna Municipal and Provincial Archives (Wiener Stadt- und Landesarchiv), Municipal Department 207 A 28 3, Copy of a disciplinary judgment (Disziplinarerkenntnis) in the case of *Fürsorgerin* Marie P., Vienna, 21.10.1932.
112 Sachße/Tennstedt (1992), p. 197.
113 Ziering (2002), p. 37.
114 Steinhauser (1994), pp. 66–67.
115 Ziering (2002), p. 46; Frey (2005); Sachße (2003), p. 240.

Bibliography

Arlt, Ilse: Die Grundlagen der Fürsorge. Vienna 1921.

Baader, Gerhard; Hofer, Veronika; Mayer, Thomas (eds.): Eugenik in Österreich. Biopolitische Strukturen von 1900 bis 1945. Vienna 2007.

Bundesamt für Statistik (ed.): Die Ergebnisse der österreichischen Volkszählung vom 2. März 1934. Bundesstaat, Tabellenheft. (= Statistik des Bundesstaates Österreich 2) Vienna 1935.

Chesnais, Jean-Claude: The Demographic Transition. Stages, Patterns, and Economic Implications. A Longitudinal Study of Sixty-Seven Countries Covering the Period 1720–1984. Oxford 1992.

Czech, Herwig: Die Inventur des Volkskörpers. Die "erbbiologische Bestandsaufnahme" im Dispositiv der NS-Rassenhygiene in Wien. In: Baader, Gerhard; Hofer, Veronika; Mayer, Thomas (eds.): Eugenik in Österreich. Biopolitische Strukturen von 1900 bis 1945. Vienna 2007, pp. 284–311.

Davies, Celia: The Health Visitor as Mother's Friend: A woman's place in public health, 1900–14. In: Social History of Medicine 1 (1988), pp. 39–59.

Dietrich-Daum, Elisabeth: Die "Wiener Krankheit". Eine Sozialgeschichte der Tuberkulose in Österreich. (= Sozial- und wirtschaftshistorische Studien 32) Vienna; Munich 2007.

Erster Österreichischer Kinderschutzkongress (ed.): Schriften des Ersten Österreichischen Kinderschutzkongresses in Wien, 1907. 3 vols. Vienna 1907.

Ertl, Ursula: Ilse Arlt – Studien zur Biographie der wenig bekannten Wissenschaftlerin und Begründerin der Fürsorgeausbildung in Österreich. Würzburg; Schweinfurt 1995.

Fehlemann, Silke; Vögele, Jörg: Frauen in der Gesundheitsfürsorge am Beginn des 20. Jahrhunderts. England und Deutschland im Vergleich. In: Lindner, Ulrike; Niehuss, Merith (eds.): Ärztinnen – Patientinnen. Frauen im deutschen und britischen Gesundheitswesen des 20. Jahrhunderts. Cologne; Weimar; Vienna 2002, pp. 23–47.

Fildes, Valerie (ed.): Women and Children First: International Maternal and Infant Welfare 1870–1945. London 1992.

Frey, Cornelia: "Respekt vor der Kreativität des Menschen". Ilse Arlt: Werk und Wirkung. (= Frauen- und Genderforschung in der Erziehungswissenschaft 1) Opladen 2005.

Gegenbauer, Viktor: Ueber soziale Hygiene. In: Gemeinde Wien (ed.): Einführung in die soziale Hygiene. Fünfzehn Aufsätze des städtischen Gesundheitsamtes für Fürsorgerinnen und Sanitätsrevisoren. Part 1–2. (Special imprint from Blätter für das Wohlfahrtswesen 29/30 nos. 279–281, 283) Vienna 1930, pp. 3–13.

Geiger, Katja: "Im Dienst der Volksgesundheit". Fürsorgerinnen bzw. Volkspflegerinnen im nationalsozialistischen Wien. In: Arias, Ingrid (ed.): Im Dienste der Volksgesundheit. Frauen – Gesundheitswesen – Nationalsozialismus. Vienna 2006, pp. 177–209.

Gemeinde Wien (ed.): Das Neue Wien. Städtewerk. Vol. 2. Vienna 1927.

Gemeinde Wien (ed.): Einführung in die soziale Hygiene. Fünfzehn Aufsätze des städtischen Gesundheitsamtes für Fürsorgerinnen und Sanitätsrevisoren. Part 1–2. (Special imprint from Blätter für das Wohlfahrtswesen 29/30 nos. 279–281, 283) Vienna 1930.

Gemeinde Wien, Magistratsabteilung 7 (ed.): Das Jugendamt der Stadt Wien. Vienna 1933.

Gottstein, Adolf: Aufgaben der Gemeinde- und der privaten Fürsorge. In: Deppe, Hans-Ulrich; Regus, Michael (eds.): Seminar: Medizin, Gesellschaft, Geschichte. Beiträge zur Entwicklungsgeschichte der Medizinsoziologie. (= suhrkamp taschenbuch wissenschaft 67) Frankfurt/Main 1975, pp. 230–241.

Gruber, Helmut: Red Vienna. Experiment in Working-Class Culture 1919–1934. New York; Oxford 1991.

Healy, Maureen: Vienna and the Fall of the Habsburg Empire. Total War and Everyday Life in World War I. Cambridge 2004.

Hecht, Dieter J.: Zwischen Feminismus und Zionismus. Die Biographie einer Wiener Jüdin. Anitta Müller-Cohen (1890–1962). (= L'Homme Schriften 15) Vienna; Cologne; Weimar 2008.

Jancsy, Peter: Jugendfürsorge in Österreich 1918–1934 unter besonderer Berücksichtigung des Wiener Wohlfahrtswesens. Vienna 1982 (unpublished thesis).

Kepplinger, Brigitte: Komunale Sozialpolitik in Linz 1938–1945. In: Mayrhofer, Fritz; Schuster, Walter (eds.): Nationalsozialismus in Linz. Vol. 1. Linz 2001, pp. 715–797.

Köstler, Marie: Die Fürsorgerin. In: Arbeiterkammer in Wien (ed.): Handbuch der Frauenarbeit in Österreich. Vienna 1930, pp. 281–294.

Kytir, Josef: Regionale Unterschiede der Säuglingssterblichkeit in Österreich. In: Mitteilungen der Österreichischen Geographischen Gesellschaft 131 (1989), pp. 47–76.

Lesky, Erna: Meilensteine der Wiener Medizin. Große Ärzte Österreichs in drei Jahrhunderten. Vienna; Munich; Berne 1981.

Lichtenberg, Elfriede: Ein Tag aus dem Leben einer Fürsorgerin. Radiovortrag gehalten am 16. März 1932. In: Österreichische Blätter für Krankenpflege und Fürsorge 8 (1932), no. 3, pp. 33–39.

Lindner, Ulrike; Niehuss, Merith (eds.): Ärztinnen – Patientinnen. Frauen im deutschen und britischen Gesundheitswesen des 20. Jahrhunderts. Cologne; Weimar; Vienna 2002.

Malleier, Elisabeth: Jüdische Frauen in Wien 1816–1938. Wohlfahrt – Mädchenbildung – Frauenarbeit. Vienna 2003.

Malleier, Elisabeth: "Making the world a better place". Welfare and politics, welfare as politics? Activities of Jewish women in Vienna before 1938. In: Aschkenas 16 (2006), pp. 261–268.

Melinz, Gerhard; Unger, Gerhard: Wohlfahrt und Krise. Wiener Kommunalpolitik 1929–1938. (= Forschungen und Beiträge zur Wiener Stadtgeschichte 29) Vienna 1996.

Melinz, Gerhard; Zimmermann, Susan: Über die Grenzen der Armenhilfe. Kommunale und staatliche Sozialpolitik in Wien und Budapest in der Doppelmonarchie. (= Materialien zur Arbeiterbewegung 60) Vienna; Zurich 1991.

Melinz, Gerhard; Zimmermann, Susan: Getrennte Wege. Wohlfahrtspolitik und gesellschaftlicher Transformationsprozess in Wien und Budapest zwischen den Weltkriegen. In: Jahrbuch des Vereins für Geschichte der Stadt Wien 50 (1994), pp. 269–315.

Mitteilungen der österreichischen Gesellschaft für Bevölkerungspolitik und Fürsorgewesen 4 (1925).

Mittermeier, Susanne Brigitte: Die Jugendfürsorgerin. Zur Professionalisierung der sozialen Kinder- und Jugendarbeit in der Wiener städtischen Fürsorge von den Anfängen bis zur Konstituierung des Berufsbildes Ende der 1920er Jahre. In: L'Homme 5 (1994), no. 2, pp. 102–120.

Moll, Leopold: Die Reichsanstalt für Mutter- und Säuglingsfürsorge in Wien. Vienna 1919.

Pirhofer, Gottfried; Sieder, Reinhard: Zur Konstitution der Arbeiterfamilie im Roten Wien. Familienpolitik, Kulturreform, Alltag und Ästhetik. In: Mitterauer, Michael; Sieder, Reinhard (eds.): Historische Familienforschung. (= suhrkamp taschenbuch wissenschaft 387) Frankfurt/Main 1982, pp. 326–368.

Pirquet, Clemens: Geburtenhäufigkeit und Säuglingssterblichkeit. In: Wiener Medizinische Wochenschrift 77 (1927), pp. 11–12.

Porter, Dorothy: Health, Civilization and the State. A history of public health from ancient to modern times. London 1999.

Report of Fürsorgerin Hermine Jakobartl from Unterweißenbach (Upper Austria). In: Mitteilungen der österreichischen Gesellschaft für Bevölkerungspolitik 4 (1925), pp. 45–47.

Rollet, Catherine: The Fight Against Infant Mortality in the Past: An International Comparison. In: Bideau, Alain; Desjardins, Bertrand; Brignoli, Héctor Pérez (eds.): Infant and Child Mortality in the Past. Oxford 1997, pp. 38–60.

Rosenhaupt, Heinrich: Die Hilfsorgane der Gesundheitsfürsorge, ihr Wirkungskreis und ihre Ausbildung. In: Gottstein, Adolf; Schlossmann, Arthur; Teleky, Ludwig (eds.): Handbuch der sozialen Hygiene und Gesundheitsfürsorge. Vol. 4. Berlin 1927, pp. 678–714.

Rozenblit, Marsha L.: The Jews of Vienna, 1867–1914. Assimilation and Identity. Albany 1983.

Sablik, Karl: Julius Tandler. Mediziner und Sozialreformer. Eine Biographie. Vienna 1983.

Sachße, Christoph: Mütterlichkeit als Beruf. Sozialarbeit, Sozialreform und Frauenbewegung 1871–1929. (= Kasseler Studien zur Sozialpolitik und Sozialpädagogik 1) 3rd ed. Weinheim; Basel; Berlin 2003.

Sachße, Christoph; Tennstedt, Florian: Der Wohlfahrtsstaat im Nationalsozialismus. (= Geschichte der Armenfürsorge in Deutschland 3) Stuttgart; Berlin; Cologne 1992.

Simon, Maria D[orothea]: Issues of Health and Welfare Policy in Austria. In: Steiner, Kurt (ed.): Tradition and Innovation in Contemporary Austria. Palo Alto 1982, pp. 109–122.

Simon, Maria Dorothea: Von Akademie zu Akademie. Zur historischen Entwicklung der Sozialarbeiterausbildung am Beispiel der Schule der Stadt Wien. In: Wilfing, Heinz (ed.): Konturen der Sozialarbeit. Ein Beitrag zu Identität und Professionalisierung der Sozialarbeit. Vienna 1993, pp. 15–24.

Simon, Maria D[orothea]: Historical Portrait: Ilse Arlt. In: European Journal of Social Work 5 (2002), no. 1, pp. 69–71.

Smekal-Huber, Erika: Seelen in Not. Tagebuchaufzeichnungen einer Fürsorgerin der Wiener Jugendgerichtshilfe. Vienna 1936.

Statistik Austria (ed.): Demographisches Jahrbuch 2006. Vienna 2007.

Steinhauser, Werner: Geschichte der Sozialarbeiterausbildung. Vienna 1994.

Stöckel, Sigrid: Säuglingsfürsorge zwischen sozialer Hygiene und Eugenik. Das Beispiel Berlins im Kaiserreich und in der Weimarer Republik. (= Veröffentlichungen der historischen Kommission zu Berlin 91) Berlin; New York 1996.

Stöckel, Sigrid: Weibliche Gesundheitsfürsorge zwischen Eigendefinition und Institutionalisierung. In: Lindner, Ulrike; Niehuss, Merith (eds.): Ärztinnen – Patientinnen. Frauen im deutschen und britischen Gesundheitswesen des 20. Jahrhunderts. Cologne; Weimar; Vienna 2002, pp. 49–71.

Tandler, Julius: Wohltätigkeit oder Fürsorge? (Wiener sozialdemokratische Bücherei). Vienna 1925.

Vallin, Jacques: Mortality in Europe from 1720 to 1914. Long-Term trends and Changes in Patterns by Age and Sex. In: Schofield, Roger; Reher, David; Bideau, Alain (eds.): The Decline of Mortality in Europe. Oxford 1991, pp. 38–67.

Weigl, Andreas: Demographischer Wandel und Modernisierung. (= Kommentare zum Historischen Atlas von Wien 1) Vienna 2000.

Weihsmann, Helmut: Das Rote Wien. Sozialdemokratische Architektur und Kommunalpolitik 1919–1934. Vienna 1985.

Wolfgruber, Gudrun: Zwischen Hilfestellung und sozialer Kontrolle. Jugendfürsorge im Roten Wien, dargestellt am Beispiel der Kindesabnahme. Vienna 1997.

Wolfgruber, Gudrun: Messbares Glück? Sozialdemokratische Konzeptionen zu Fürsorge und Familie im Wien der 1920er Jahre. In: L'Homme 10 (1999), no. 2, pp. 277–294.

Ziering, Gabriele: 90 Jahre Jugendamt Ottakring 1913 bis 2003. Von der Berufsvormundschaft zur Jugendwohlfahrt der MAG ELF. Vienna 2002.

The medical mission of British child guidance 1918–1950: Theory and practice

John Stewart

Introduction – What was child guidance?

In this essay we focus on a non-medical professional – the psychiatric social worker (PSW) – in a movement which had explicitly medical, and indeed scientific, pretensions, British child guidance. The period covered is from the 1920s, when child guidance established itself in Britain, down to the immediate post-Second World War era when it was embedded in the emerging 'welfare state' by way of legislation passed in the mid 1940s – in particular, the Education Acts but also the National Health Service Acts. As in the United States, where the movement originated in the aftermath of World War One, British child guidance was in the first instance largely financed by the American philanthropic body, the Commonwealth Fund of New York. Legislative recognition resulted from both a growing demand for child guidance services and the experience of the wartime evacuation of children from major urban centres.[1] It also embodied thereby a shift from essentially voluntary to essentially state provision.[2] Focussing on psychiatric social workers raises important issues about the actual content of child guidance and of the role of non-medical professionals in purportedly medical movements.

There are three contextual points which need emphasis. First, in the interwar era child guidance was part of the broader, international, movement for mental hygiene – indeed child guidance was the central component of the Commonwealth Fund's English [sic] Mental Hygiene Program.[3] The co-ordinating body for British child guidance, the Child Guidance Council, was closely allied to the National Council for Mental Hygiene and other similar bodies with which it was eventually to merge in the 1940s.[4] Mental hygiene saw itself as a form of preventive medicine and, as such, the mental health equivalent of the public health movement of the nineteenth century. The claims of mental hygiene had been given impetus by the impact and outcomes of the First World War; and, associated with this, the increasing influence of the so-called 'new psychology'.[5] Taken together, these appeared to substanti-

---

1   See Welshman (1998); and, for the particular case of Scotland, Stewart/Welshman (2006).
2   For recent discussions of British child guidance, including the historiography, see Stewart (2006); Stewart (2009). On the shift from voluntary to public provision, see Stewart (2011). For American child guidance see Jones (1999).
3   On mental hygiene see Thomson (1995).
4   For the discussions around better co-ordination in the field of mental health and welfare see The Feversham Committee (1939).
5   On psychology in twentieth century Britain see Thomson (2006).

ate the power of the subconscious and irrational components of the human mind as well as suggesting that the very nature of modern life could have deleterious effects on mental health. As one prominent participant in British mental hygiene put it, the 'increasing speed of life made possible by scientific progress is tending to produce breakdown and strain'.[6] For the child guidance movement what this suggested was that even the most 'normal' child might, in the course of its emotional and psychological development, experience 'maladjustment'. To put it another way, the whole child population was potentially under threat and so had to be carefully monitored.[7] This maladjustment might manifest itself in a range of ways, from bed-wetting through abnormal sexual behaviour through mild forms of delinquency to excessive shyness.

As will be evident, the clinical precision of a category such as 'shyness' is open to considerable question, an issue we return to below. Nonetheless not to address problems such as these would lead to unhappiness and instability for the child, both now and in later adulthood; the child's family; and society as a whole. The maladjusted child had thus to be readjusted and reintegrated both personally and socially and as I argue elsewhere this language of adjustment, instability, and integration has to be seen in a much wider scientific, social scientific, and cultural context wherein instability seemed to be a fundamental constituent of the human and natural condition.[8] Both parents and children therefore needed help to navigate what one psychiatrist involved in the movement described as the 'Dangerous Age of Childhood'.[9] Once again, this highlights the preventive medicine role mental hygiene and child guidance ascribed to themselves.

Second, and as noted, the wartime evacuation of children from threatened urban areas provided further impetus to the child guidance movement. Evacuation appeared to expose the problems of, in particular, urban working-class children; and provided a 'laboratory' for the study of children separated from their parents for investigators both in Britain and further afield.[10] As the psychiatrist John Bowlby told Board of Education officials in September 1939 – that is, as the evacuation process was getting under way – the prospect of large numbers of children 'being separated from their mothers for a period of as long as three years raised very big problems and there was a danger of large scale social maladaptation'.[11] Bowlby had undertaken part of his training at the London Child Guidance Clinic, had based some of his early research publications on this experience, and was soon internationally famous for his work

---

6 The Feversham Committee (1939), p. x.
7 On the issue of 'normalcy' in childhood see Turmel (2008), passim, and Stewart (forthcoming 2011). On the idea of monitoring, see Armstrong (1995).
8 Stewart (2009).
9 Gordon (1938).
10 On the latter point see, for example, the study by the New York-based Wolf (1945).
11 The National Archives, ED 50/273, Board of Education: Interview Memorandum, M481/33 (4), 'Behaviour Problems Among Evacuated Children', 30th September 1939.

on 'attachment theory'.[12] Another psychiatrist and one of the founders of the East End Jewish clinic, Emanuel Miller, told a child guidance conference in 1941 that if the war had 'necessitated vast evacuation of children' this 'uprooting and transplantation' would nonetheless aid in the study of 'social and psychological phenomena as they have never been studied before. It is from such studies that we will draw wisdom for a future mental hygiene plan.'[13] Such perceptions, which went beyond psychiatrists and civil servants, prompted a range of bodies, official and unofficial, to press for greater child guidance provision. So, for instance, a Scottish women's group, reviewing evacuation and its consequences, argued that child guidance 'should be extensively developed, as providing in many cases a solution to the problem child's difficulties'.[14]

Third, child guidance placed considerable emphasis on its medical, indeed scientific, credentials. Although this was highly contested, and although child guidance was not the first movement concerned with children's welfare to make such a claim, for present purposes child guidance saw itself as a form of psychiatric medicine at a point when psychiatry itself was seeking to be identified and integrated with scientific medicine.[15] The locus of child guidance was the clinic where the child patient encountered members of three professions – psychiatry, psychology, and psychiatric social work. As this implies, child guidance took an holistic approach, arguing that the child had to be seen as a totality, a totality which fore-grounded the emotional environment in which he or she lived. So although note was made of factors such as the child patient's physical surroundings, family history, and educational progress, essentially what was key was the nature of the child-parent relationship. This approach was largely derived from the theory of 'psychobiology' propounded by the American psychiatrist Adolf Meyer, hugely influential on British and American child guidance and British psychiatry in general.[16] And while much was made of this 'teamwork' approach it was, as in many other branches of 'scientific' medicine, hierarchical teamwork wherein the medically-trained psychiatrist took the lead role.[17] Such a scientific, medical approach was necessary precisely because, so it was claimed, it was pointless, indeed dangerous, to treat the symptoms of maladjustment alone. Rather, the underlying aetiology of the disease – the language of child guidance was suffused with that of medicine – had to be understood. An appropriate diagnosis could then take place, and treatment prescribed. Taken as a whole, this was the American, or medical, model of child guidance.

12   For a recent discussion of Bowlby see Mayhew (2006).
13   Miller (1941), p. 19.
14   The Scottish Women's Group on Public Welfare (1944), p. 42.
15   Stewart (2009).
16   Stewart (forthcoming 2011).
17   On medical teamwork see Sturdy/Cooter (1998).

Child guidance in practice – The role of the psychiatric social worker

How, then, did this work out in practice? A child presenting symptoms of mal-adjustment would, as we have seen, encounter members of three distinct pro-fessions at the child guidance clinic. The lead figure, the psychiatrist, was re-sponsible for physical and mental examination and, ultimately, for determin-ing diagnosis and treatment. The psychologist administered various forms of mental testing. The third professional, and the one on which this paper fo-cuses, was the PSW and before examining her role we need to say something briefly about how this profession emerged.[18]

Psychiatric social work emerged in the aftermath of the First World War, in the first instance in the USA. Training in psychiatric social work was ini-tially offered at Smith College in 1918 with other training centres, for example at the Institute for Child Guidance in New York, emerging thereafter.[19] Re-porting on a visit to view American child guidance centres in the late 1920s, once again funded by the Commonwealth Fund, a British social worker noted that the 'rapid growth and development of psychiatric social work in America during the last ten years is one of the most striking facts in the history of Men-tal Hygiene work'.[20] As Jones remarks of America the 'child guidance social worker belonged to a new breed, with intellectual ties to dynamic psychiatry as well as roots in nineteenth-century altruism'.[21] In general terms this was also true of Britain, although as we shall see there were important differences in approach in the British case. And while PSWs from the outset certainly en-gaged with groups other than children it was nonetheless with child guidance that it was especially associated and most visible, in both the US and Britain.

The first British training course in psychiatric social work – the Diploma in Mental Health – was initiated at the London School of Economics (LSE) in 1929, with the Commonwealth Fund again providing the bulk of the financial resources.[22] In the inter-war period the course was successful in attracting stu-dents not only from the United Kingdom but also from other European coun-tries. So, for instance, in 1934 it was noted that the course had been recognised as suitable for training Dutch social workers. The following year applicants from abroad came from the Netherlands, Germany, Norway, Sweden, Swit-

---

18 For an analysis of a closely-related profession, which raises similar issues to those dis-cussed here, see Nottingham/Dougall (2007).

19 Witmer (1930) – the author wrote a number of important works on American child guid-ance; Swift (1934).

20 University of Liverpool, Papers of Professor Sir Cyril Burt, D.191/20/1/9, Miss St Clair Townsend, 'Report on Psychiatric Social Work', n. d. but late 1920s, p. 1.

21 Jones (1999), p. 78.

22 British Library of Political and Economic Science, Archives of the London School of Eco-nomics and Political Science (hereafter BLPES), Central Filing Registry/514/1/A, letter, 31st January 1929, Child Guidance Council to William Beveridge, LSE. For Britain more generally see Stewart (2007). See also the account of the emergence of British psychiatric social workers by one of its early practitioners: Timms (1964).

zerland, and potentially China.[23] In September 1939, meanwhile, there were two Dutch, one South African, and one Australian as students on the course, supplemented by refugees from Germany and Czechoslovakia.[24] Relatively small as these numbers were, nonetheless students from overseas were important in bringing or consolidating child guidance principles and practice to their own countries and, more indirectly, in thereby importing the 'American' model.[25]

By 1950 there were two other courses, at the Universities of Edinburgh and Manchester, further evidence of the growing demand for child guidance services.[26] The LSE course began a process of professionalising British social work and indeed psychiatric social work regarded itself, down to its abolition as a specialism in the 1970s, as in the vanguard of the profession. Timms remarked in the 1960s, for example, that its professional association was 'perhaps the strongest, although by no means the largest, of the professional social work organizations'.[27] So, as I have argued elsewhere, psychiatric social work saw itself as 'qualitatively different from other forms of social work'.[28] From a different angle, Nottingham suggests, in his discussion of what he describes as 'insecure professionals', that such occupational groups 'have always sought to improve their condition by trying to emulate the established (professions)', for example through training.[29] This sense of creating a distinctive professional identity is captured in the case of psychiatric social work by the aims of its professional body, the Association of Psychiatric Social Workers (ASPW), an organisation which clearly modelled itself on its American counterpart. These aims included the raising and maintaining of professional standards; the encouragement of the 'employment of fully trained workers at adequate salaries'; and 'promoting and facilitating research'.[30]

In terms of child guidance practice the PSW's responsibility was to observe and gather information on the child and its family, both at the clinic itself and through home visits. In each of these situations the child might be observed as well as spoken to directly, as might other members of the family, the aim being to assess the emotional relationships prevailing within the do-

---

23 BLPES, Minutes of School Committees/16/8, Mental Health Course Consultative Committee, 8th June 1934 and 5th November 1935.

24 BLPES, Central Filing Registry/514/2/D, letter, 12th September 1939, Professor Carr-Saunders, LSE, to Barry Smith, Commonwealth Fund.

25 On the introduction of child guidance to the Netherlands see Oosterhuis (2005), pp.79–83, where he notes, inter alia, the growing adoption of the American model in the 1930s.

26 Ministry of Health, 'Report of the Committee on Social Workers in the Mental Health Services', Cmd.8260, London, Her Majesty's Stationery Office, 1951, pp.10ff.

27 Timms (1964), p.6.

28 Stewart (2009).

29 Nottingham (2007), p.462.

30 Modern Records Centre, University of Warwick, Archives of the Association of Psychiatric Social Workers (hereafter MRC), MSS.378/APSW/P/2/2, The Association of Psychiatric Social Workers, 'Report for the Year 1936 (with Foreword on the years 1930–35)', p.5.

mestic environment. These observations and analyses were then conveyed to the clinic case conferences and so informed the psychiatrist's diagnosis and proposed treatment. The outcome of these deliberations was then transmitted, again by the psychiatric social worker, to the child and its family with the PSW having the task of ensuring that the prescribed treatment was duly carried out.

Clearly, then, the psychiatric social worker had a crucial role in child guidance and so her professional training was, purportedly, crucial. William Moodie, psychiatrist and Director of the British movement's focal point, the London Child Guidance Clinic, remarked that the PSW's investigation of the home was a matter of 'scientific observation' and not just simple question and answer.[31] Another psychiatrist, R.G. Gordon, argued that the individual trained in psychiatric social work could, among other things, 'avoid the pitfalls with which the path of the well-meaning "common-sense" worker is so liberally strewn'.[32] In an early edition of the *British Journal of Psychiatric Social Work*, launched by the ASPW shortly after the Second World War, one of the profession's leading supporters and key member of the child guidance movement, the psychiatrist Douglas MacCalman, suggested that PSWs 'must be creative and stimulate others to creative activity, which must be turned first against material and external challenges, and then towards the self in an effort to attain inner harmony'.[33]

Unsurprisingly, PSWs themselves emphasised their specialised training and the unique insights it afforded to individual cases and, indeed, more generally. Two leading practitioners argued that there was an 'element of reciprocity between social work and psychiatry' and a 'need of each profession for what the other has to give'. More specifically, what the specially-trained PSW brought to this relationship was 'a perceptiveness to the "body social"' and the profession was thus more than simply 'ancillary' to psychiatry. So, for instance, the influence of Freud and psychoanalysis was of 'special importance [...] for social workers who were to train for work with the mentally ill and maladjusted'.[34] Clearly, and in line with our earlier observation about its self-appointed leading role in social work, psychiatric social work saw itself as being about more than just information gathering.

As Timms put it, one characteristic of child guidance work was that social workers 'were implicitly or explicitly concerned for the first time with human behaviour and relationships <u>as their primary function</u>'.[35] Or, as another PSW remarked in the late 1930s, she and her colleagues not only used their 'training and experience' to evaluate the facts and understand their significance. They also, through contact with the patient's family and friends, had 'to inter-

---

31 University of Manchester, John Rylands Library, Store (Med.Pam.2)/87.29: Moodie, William: Child Guidance by Team Work. London 1931, p.3.
32 Gordon (1939).
33 MacCalman (1948), p.94.
34 Ashdown/Brown (1953), pp. 11, 12, 15.
35 Timms (1964), p.4, my emphasis.

pret to them the illness, the treatment, the psychological and emotional tangles in which both patient and family seem to be tied up'. In so doing, of course, the PSW had to 'keep her own attitude objective, so that she can present the situation in its true perspective'.[36] In other words, as a result of their particular training and skills, PSWs were active participants in both diagnosis and treatment and this was seen as a crucial refinement of their role in the course of the 1930s.[37] Again, it is possible to discern American influence here. In the late 1920s a PSW prominent in the US child guidance movement wrote that because 'emotional difficulties' required social as well as medical analysis the 'psychiatric social worker takes on an important part with the psychiatrist and the psychologist in the study of the patient and his environment'.[38] Reviewing the history of psychiatric social work training in the early 1950s a government report noted that from early on it had been understood that a 'high standard of clinical practice was essential to the success of the training'.[39] The use of the word 'clinical' again suggests the medical credentials which psychiatric social work claimed.

Here, then, we appear to have a particular profession – psychiatric social work – which is part of an explicitly medical project – child guidance. The PSW was, so it was argued, highly trained and, implicitly at least, less of a subordinate to the psychiatrist than a co-worker with an almost equally vital role in the diagnosis and treatment of child mental maladjustment. This was deemed acceptable or even desirable, and not simply on the grounds of training and professional standards. Most child guidance psychiatrists openly acknowledged that they only had time to see their patients very briefly (and the patient's family even less) and that it was the social workers who had by far the most contact with the child patients and their families. This could be further justified by child guidance's holistic approach whereby the patient's environment – which generally meant the emotional landscape of the home – was crucial in creating any maladjustment from which the child suffered.[40]

Embracing these points MacCalman told an audience in 1949 that the 'debt which psychiatrists owe to ancillary workers must be recognized'. In future groups like social workers must be used 'so that they will be able to do a great deal of the work now undertaken by psychiatrists. In this way we may be able to husband our resources, while maintaining our efficiency.'[41] Moodie, meanwhile, described the trained psychiatric social worker as 'an invaluable asset in treatment'. She could interpret the psychiatrist's findings for the par-

---

36   Lane (1939), p. 133.
37   See also Stewart (2007).
38   Odencrantz (1929), p. 264.
39   Ministry of Health, 'Report of the Committee on Social Workers in the Mental Health Services', Cmd. 8260, London, Her Majesty's Stationery Office, 1951, p. 12.
40   In certain circumstances, for instance when dealing with evacuated children, PSWs seem to have been virtually in sole charge. See Kanter (2000), p. 248.
41   'Discussion of the Development of Psychiatry within the National Health Service'. In: *Proceedings of the Royal Society of Medicine* 42 (1949), p. 365.

ents which had the benefit of saving the time of the clinic's medical staff. More than this, though, parents were often more inclined to accept advice from a PSW whereas 'the didactic prescription of the doctor is unheeded'.[42] Recalling his early training at the London Child Guidance Clinic, Bowlby commented on the contribution of 'an exceptionally able group of psychiatric social workers to whom I have always felt very deeply indebted'. These included Robina Addis who had, Bowlby claimed, 'no qualms about putting conceited medicals in their place'.[43]

Problems with psychiatric social work

Of course, this was not as unproblematic as proponents of child guidance might have imagined or desired. Here I focus on three issues: the contested nature of child guidance; PSW training; and, in particular, the actual practice of psychiatric social work. First, then, the contested nature of child guidance.[44] Challenges to child guidance came from a range of sources. Some within psychiatry, notably supporters of Melanie Klein and of Anna Freud, argued against its holistic approach, stressing instead the internal workings of the child's mind. Psychologists, meanwhile, claimed that child maladjustment was a behavioural rather than a medical problem which could be dealt with by psychologists and teachers. This was particularly true in Scotland where educational psychology was strong and where the American/medical model of child guidance gained little purchase. These various challenges were both mutually antagonistic while, implicitly or explicitly, questioning the need for psychiatric social workers, and particularly their quasi-medical role. Indeed it is notable that some social workers and psychiatric social workers themselves questioned the notion that their profession was 'medical' or 'scientific', preferring instead to stress the 'art' of social work which derived from experience, intuition, and empathy – a very traditional approach.[45]

Second, there is the question of how PSWs were actually trained. We have seen that the instigation of the Diploma in Mental Health 1929 was a crucial step towards professionalizing social work in general, and that psychiatric social work thereby led the way in this process. Students were usually expected to have some sort of qualification and, equally important, existing social work experience. So, for instance, of the cohort which qualified in 1936 44% had degrees, with the remainder having degrees and/or Certificates in Social Sci-

---

42 Wellcome Library for the History and Understanding of Medicine (hereafter Wellcome), Robina Scott Addis Papers, PP/ADD/C.3/5: Moodie, William: 'Child Guidance and the Schools', pamphlet reprinted from *Head Teachers Review*, February 1931, pp. 9–10.

43 Wellcome, John Bowlby Papers, PP/BOW/C.5, copy of *The Child Guidance Trust: Newsletter No. 3* (June 1987), pp. 1–2.

44 For fuller discussions of these points see Stewart (2009); Stewart (2006); and Stewart (2007).

45 For the broad picture, see Timms (1997).

ence.[46] On admission, as the account of Ashdown and Clement Brown explained, students were introduced to the 'discoveries which psychology and psychiatry, including analytic concepts, have brought to bear upon the problems of human behaviour'. This enabled a 'further understanding of the healthy and the sick individual, how personality normally develops and how its development comes to be disturbed' thereby allowing for 'an introduction to clinical psychiatry'.[47] There is little doubt that the LSE training was far more comprehensive than anything which preceded it and there can be little doubt that this specialist education contributed strongly to the collective identity of psychiatric social work.

Having said that, the course did only last ten months. During this time the student undertook a placement for three days each week during which she would gain experience of around five to eight cases. Classroom teaching was thus confined to the other two days and included topics such as psychiatry, psychology, mental hygiene, and social case work.[48] This was clearly demanding enough. But it is difficult to envisage that any particular subject could be gone into in any depth and indeed this was something recognised by some of the LSE staff themselves. In 1939, the psychologist Lucy Fildes wrote to the relevant academic committee expressing the difficulty of 'planning an adequate syllabus in the basic facts and concepts of psychology' for such a short course.[49] Even proponents of psychiatric social work such as Ashdown and Clement Brown, while keen to assert professional status, admitted that the training they described took place within 'the limits of a one year course'.[50] Overall, it is hard to disagree with the historian of American social work, Roy Lubove. As he puts it, how in the last resort might one distinguish between psychiatric social workers, psychiatrists, and psychotherapists? For Lubove, the answer was simple: 'the social worker's inferior training'.[51]

This raises the questions of both the content of psychiatric social work training and its relationship to the other child guidance professions. It is revealing that while the rhetoric of teamwork was consistently stressed by all child guidance professionals, this nonetheless remained a hierarchical relationship. Psychiatrists, as we have seen, often fulsomely praised PSWs and their work. But occasionally another face revealed itself. The eminent psychiatrist D.K. Henderson told a medical audience as early as the mid 1920s that psychiatric social work demanded 'very definite and careful training'. It should, however, 'only be practised by those who have had a specialised

---

46 BLPES, Central Filing Registry/514/2/B, letter, 30th July 1936, CM Lloyd, LSE, to Barry Smith, Commonwealth Fund.
47 Ashdown/Brown (1953), p. 21.
48 See MRC, MSS.378/APSW/P/12/20, which contains materials relating to the LSE course which have been selected and synthesised here.
49 BLPES, Minutes of School Committees/16/5, Mental Health Course Academic Sub-Committee, Minutes 18th May 1939.
50 Ashdown/Brown (1953), p. 21.
51 Lubove (1965), p. 117.

course, and <u>only under medical instruction</u>'. There was, he continued, 'far too much tendency now for both social workers and for psychologists to invade the medical field, and, acting on their own, they are apt to be a source of danger rather than any great help'.[52] Even more robustly, a psychiatrist at the Liverpool Child Guidance Clinic remarked that the PSW 'can do no more than maintain supervision in the home, ensuring as far as possible that the management of the child and the attitudes of parents and associates are reasonable'. It was the psychiatrist's responsibility to 'understand the child and to bring about a solution of the problem'.[53] Here then were forthright assertions of the primacy of the medical profession and, especially in the latter case, of the medical dominance of the American/medical model of child guidance.

Third, in the light of the two preceding points what was it psychiatric social workers actually did with their child patients and just how 'medical' was this? This is not easy to unpick, as case notes are rare and published accounts by psychiatric social workers concerning their work tended to reinforce the professional self-identity which they sought. But there are some case records extant along with other accounts which illuminate, often unwittingly, the framework and limitations of PSW intervention.

Case studies – Child patients at home and in the clinic

Beatrice Robinson, psychiatric social worker at the Jewish East End Child Guidance Clinic, shared some of her experiences with readers of the popular journal *Mother and Child*. She noted, for instance, the case of a young boy whose pilfering coincided with the absence of his father from the family home. The latter had a number of admirable qualities – he was described, for example, as 'a most affectionate father' – but was, nonetheless, 'an incurably erratic personality'. During the father's absences the child's mother, an 'ultra-sensitive and reserved woman' nonetheless devoted to her child, was effectively left destitute. The PSW had, however, gained the woman's confidence and advised her on how to handle the family's financial affairs. Ultimately, though, this was a case where 'no fundamental change can be hoped for'. Rather, the psychiatric social worker's role was to be 'one influence amongst many other extraneous influences at work' while the passage of time ameliorated the husband's fecklessness.[54] In many respects this was a perfectly straightforward social work case in the sense that while the child's motivations were ascribed to his father's behaviour nonetheless the 'solutions' to the family's problems followed a fairly 'traditional' social work line – counselling the mother about financial matters and how best to deal with her husband. But some of the

52 Henderson (1925), p. 291 – my emphasis.
53 University of Liverpool, Archives and Special Collections, EX 65:36, The Liverpool Child Guidance Council, 'Report for the Year 1936', Liverpool, The Liverpool Child Guidance Council, presumably 1937, p. 18.
54 Robinson (1933), pp. 353–354.

more imprecise, at least in clinical terms, concepts often utilised in child guid-ance are also present here – for instance in noting the sensitivity of the mother and the affectionate nature of the father.

A more complicated case can be found in the example of a London girl referred in the early 1930s for stealing and truancy. She was dealt with by the PSW already encountered, Robina Addis, who was in many ways an exem-plar of her profession being involved in, for instance, a serious and important research project on bed-wetting.[55] In the case of the truant girl Addis's initial input included empirical information on the child's accommodation and pa-rental income. But more impressionistic and normative material was also in-troduced. The recently-widowed father was described as 'easy going, affec-tionate and kindly'. The patient's elder sister deeply resented the former's lack of involvement in housework while the baby of the family 'gets all the petting'. A further home visit revealed that the father was 'vaguely distressed' about the patient and concerned about her mixing with boys. The girl appeared 'ex-tremely wayward and irresponsible' while further note was made of the spoil-ing of the youngest child. So what we find is an uneasy mixture of extremely imprecise, descriptive, language such as 'easy going' and 'vaguely distressed' alongside more obviously factual material. To add a further dimension to this, the same PSW in other cases again used normative comments such as 'whole atmosphere in house is stiff and drab' alongside phrases such as 'strong ego-drive' and 'libidinal urge'. So we have another layer of discourse – clinical, or at least purportedly clinical. To return to our original case it might seem espe-cially ironic that after all the input from the psychiatrist and the psychologist as well as the PSW what was finally agreed was that the patient and her family could only be helped in 'practical ways'. Consequently, various traditional social work measures were undertaken – for example, enquiring of a particu-lar charity whether it could help with clothing.[56]

More complicated still was the case of a young boy referred in early 1933 to the Edinburgh Catholic Child Guidance Clinic due to his mother's inability to control his behaviour and his lack of control in his toilet habits. Detailed notes were taken of the PSW's interviews with the child and with his mother. The latter, 'Italian by birth', was apparently in poor physical condition but nonetheless demonstrated 'considerable intelligence and insight' into the child's problems and seemed 'genuinely fond of him and anxious to do her best'. The child himself was illegitimate and had for the first two years of his life been boarded with an old woman who, it was claimed by the mother, 'knew nothing about children'. The child was slow in developing physically and exhibited from the outset various nervous traits, for instance fear of the dark. He was quarrelsome, dishonest, and untruthful, again by the mother's account. The PSW found the child shy and nervous, answering her questions

55 Addis (1935).
56 Wellcome, Robina Scott Addis Papers, PP/ADD/C.1/8 and PP/ADD/C.1/9 – these records have been accessed on the condition and understanding that any citations are anonymised.

in a whisper. The key problem, though, was the child's relationship with his step-father. The latter effectively refused to acknowledge the former's existence with the boy telling his fellow school pupils that 'as soon as he is big enough he is going to leave home because his Daddy does not want him'. The husband, who drank and gambled and kept his wife short of money, had not worked since his marriage and the child's mother blamed him for her child's difficulties.

Summing up, the interview notes highlighted two points. First, the physical neglect of the child during his first two years which had at least in part contributed to his phobias. Second, the child's treatment by his step-father. This had produced feelings of inferiority for which the child 'tries to compensate by defiance and negativism'. Among the manifestations of this were his poor toilet habits and his dishonesty. While a fuller investigation of the patient's 'mental and emotional life' would have to be undertaken – presumably by the psychiatrist – provisional assessment suggested the need either to alter the step-father's attitude or, if this proved difficult, to move the child into a 'more sympathetic and kindly atmosphere' while ensuring that he did not feel he had been driven out of his home. Crucial here was that the mother be encouraged to take 'an affectionate interest in his welfare'.[57]

As in the preceding case, the PSW here is clearly attempting to employ her analytical and clinical training in an attempt to comprehend and convey to the rest of the child guidance team the emotional (and physical) landscape of the child patient's environment in what was clearly a difficult, complex, and distressing family situation. What would appear to be perfectly plausible, psychiatrically-based, explanations are put forward for the child's behaviour and emotional and psychological state. Nonetheless it is difficult not to see a judgemental undertow to, in particular, the assessment of the step-father and, more obliquely, the child's illegitimacy. Indeed there is a common theme in the three cases cited relating to the role of parents. For the British child guidance movement parenting must be neither too indulgent nor too strict – an 'affectionate interest' was the ideal. It helped too, of course, if both parents were actually present in the household. Returning to our third case we again encounter comprehensible and yet vague notions such as shyness in the child and anxiety in the mother.

Conclusion – The limitations of child guidance and psychiatric social work

Of course on one level it is unreasonable, even anachronistic, to criticise psychiatric social work for problems of language and definition. So while, for ex-

---

57 Scottish Catholic Archives, Edinburgh, DE 125/52, Edinburgh Child 12 – these records have been accessed on the condition and understanding that any citations are anonymised.

ample, words such as 'shyness' lack precision they nonetheless do succeed in conveying a particular mood or characteristic. But the whole issue of how to describe and evaluate emotional states was a deeply troubling issue for the child guidance movement as a whole in the period under consideration. Indeed it was a concern which exercised some of the leading child guidance psychiatrists such as MacCalman and Moodie. In the late 1940s, for instance, MacCalman noted that the 'growth of character and personality' was the most important 'mode of development'. Emotional development was, though, 'subtle, capricious and ephemeral' and without 'exact methods of measurement and comparison'.[58]

British child guidance was, furthermore, for the most part anxious to avoid any association with psychoanalysis and, relatedly, with an over-emphasis on child sexuality. Moodie, for example, claimed that the 'psycho-analytic method is never employed in a Child Guidance Clinic' (emphasis in original). Rather, the discussions between psychiatrist and child patient 'need only follow the lines of an ordinary commonsense conversation'.[59] Given such pragmatism it is thus unsurprising that PSWs likewise might incline to a 'traditional' social work approach, a strategy reinforced by the limited nature of their training and their place in the child guidance hierarchy. In passing, it is instructive to note the more 'rigorous' – or at least psychoanalytically informed – approach to psychiatry in child guidance social work adopted in some other countries and involving psychiatric social workers. This was the case, for instance, in the home of child guidance, the United States; and countries to which it was 'exported', such as the Netherlands.[60] Indeed it is instructive to compare British discussions of psychiatric social work with, most notably, their American counterparts with the latter placing much more emphasis on 'theory' rather than 'practice'.[61] Such approaches lead one commentator to identify the shift from 'child guidance' to 'child psychiatry' in the United States as occurring as early as the 1930s.[62]

In turn, this suggests the limitations, at least in a 'medical' sense, of both psychiatric social work and child guidance in Britain during the period under consideration. To put it at its simplest, child guidance was a movement which claimed an overtly medical, even scientific, approach. There were, undoubtedly, medical dimensions to child guidance theory and practice and we have seen, in the particular case of psychiatric social work, interpretations based at least in part on psychiatric theory. Nonetheless and almost certainly unwittingly, logistical constraints combined with an emphasis on seeing the child in its total environment resulted in the focus of attention being, in essence, the

58 MacCalman (1947), pp. v, vii. This point is developed in more depth in Stewart (forthcoming 2011).
59 University of Manchester, John Rylands Library, Store (Med.Pam.2)/87.29: Moodie, William: Child Guidance by Team Work. London 1931, p. 5.
60 Jones (1999), ch. 3; Oosterhuis (2005).
61 See, for example, French (1940).
62 Smuts (2006), ch. 12.

child and its family in their domestic setting. It was in this context that the PSW both engaged with the child patient's problem; then conveyed her observations back to the clinic so as to inform diagnosis and treatment. Both diagnosis and treatment might well be informed by psychiatric theory, but in practice much of the latter appears to have involved more 'traditional' social work concerns and approaches, the professional training of psychiatric social workers notwithstanding.

We noted earlier Nottingham's work on 'insecure professionals'. Nottingham further suggests that such professionals 'operated at the point where state and society met the individual'. 'They were', he continues, 'messengers of obligation, witnesses to misfortune, and, so often, administrators of society's zero sums. They rarely had much influence over the creation of the rules they applied though they could bend them.'[63] This is clearly not an unproblematic formulation. But it does, I would suggest, offer an insight into professions such as psychiatric social work. Here was a body of workers which, as we have seen, sought professional status and were seen as essential to the child guidance team in which it was they who, essentially, undertook the largest volume of work. But their situation was also, for example, one of subordination to a much more highly trained profession – medicine – while their mode of actual practice was often pragmatic and practical rather than driven by the psychiatric theory they conscientiously but briefly studied during their training. More broadly, the PSW experience in child guidance raises issues about exactly how 'medical' child guidance was in this era in addition to illustrating the problematic status of such 'subordinate' groups in medical movements and practice.

Bibliography

Addis, Robina S.: A Statistical Study of Nocturnal Enuresis. In: Archives of Diseases in Childhood 10 (1935), pp. 169–178.

Armstrong, David: The Rise of Surveillance Medicine. In: Sociology of Health and Illness 17 (1995), pp. 393–404.

Ashdown, Margaret; Brown, S. Clement: Social Service and Mental Health: An Essay on Psychiatric Social Workers. London 1953.

The Feversham Committee: The Voluntary Mental Health Services: The Report of the Feversham Committee. London 1939.

French, Lois Meredith: Psychiatric Social Work. New York 1940.

Gordon, Ronald Grey: Address to Mothers: The Dangerous Age of Childhood. In: Mother and Child 9 (1938), pp. 80–85.

Gordon, Ronald Grey: Foreword. In: Gordon, Ronald Grey (ed.): A Survey of Child Psychiatry. London 1939.

Henderson, David Kennedy: Some Preventive Aspects of Psychiatric Work. In: Glasgow Medical Journal 103 (1925), pp. 283–291.

Jones, Kathleen: Taming the Troublesome Child: American Families, Child Guidance, and the Limits of Psychiatric Authority. Cambridge, Mass. 1999.

63 Nottingham (2007), p. 469.

Kanter, Joel: The Untold Story of Clare and Donald Winnicott: How Social Work Influenced Modern Psychoanalysis. In: Clinical Social Work Journal 28 (2000), pp. 245–261.

Lane, M.A.: The Place of the Social Worker in Mental Health. In: Mental Hygiene 5 (1939), pp. 132–136.

Lubove, Roy: The Professional Altruist: The Emergence of Social Work as a Career, 1880–1930. Cambridge, Mass. 1965.

MacCalman, Douglas: Foreword. In: Bowley, Agatha H. (ed.): The Natural Development of the Child. Edinburgh 1947, pp. 5–8.

MacCalman, Douglas R.: Sweet Are the Uses of Adversity. In: British Journal of Psychiatric Social Work 2 (1948), pp. 87–94.

Mayhew, Ben: Between Love and Aggression: The Politics of John Bowlby. In: History of the Human Sciences 19 (2006), pp. 19–35.

Miller, Emanuel: The Future of the Mental Hygiene of Children. In: The Child Guidance Council (ed.): The Future of Child Guidance in Relation to War Experience. London 1941, pp. 18–24.

Nottingham, Chris: The Rise of the Insecure Professionals. In: International Review of Social History 52 (2007), pp. 445–475.

Nottingham, Chris; Dougall, Rona: A Close and Practical Association with the Medical Profession: Scottish Medical Social Workers and Social Medicine, 1940–1975. In: Medical History 51 (2007), pp. 309–336.

Odencrantz, Louise C.: The Social Worker in Family, Medical and Psychiatric Social Work. New York 1929.

Oosterhuis, Harry: Insanity and Other Discomforts: A Century of Outpatient Psychiatry and Mental Health Care in the Netherlands, 1900–2000. In: Gijswijt-Hofstra, Marijke et al (eds.): Psychiatric Cultures Compared: Psychiatry and Mental Health Care in the Twentieth Century. Amsterdam 2005, pp. 73–102.

Robinson, Beatrice H.: The Social Approach to Problems of Child Guidance. In: Mother and Child 10 (1933), pp. 353–355.

The Scottish Women's Group on Public Welfare: Our Scottish Towns: Evacuation and the Social Future. Edinburgh 1944.

Smuts, Alice Boardman: Science in the Service of Children, 1893–1935. New Haven 2006.

Stewart, John: Child Guidance in Interwar Scotland: International Influences and Domestic Concerns. In: Bulletin of the History of Medicine 80 (2006), pp. 513–539.

Stewart, John: 'I Thought You Would Want to Come and See His Home': Child Guidance and Psychiatric Social Work in Interwar Britain. In: Jackson, Mark (ed.): Health and the Modern Home. London 2007, pp. 111–127.

Stewart, John: The Scientific Claims of British Child Guidance, 1918–1950. In: British Journal for the History of Science 42 (2009), pp. 407–432.

Stewart, John: Child Guidance in Britain, 1927–1951: From Voluntarism to the Welfare State. In: Gosling, George; Penn, Alison; Rochester, Colin; Zimmeck, Meta (eds.): Tragedy or Farce? Voluntary Action in Historical Perspective. Brighton 2011.

Stewart, John: 'The Dangerous Age of Childhood': Child Guidance and the 'Normal' Child in Great Britain, 1920–1950. In: Paedagogica Historica (forthcoming 2011).

Stewart, John; Welshman, John: The Evacuation of Children in Wartime Scotland: Culture, Behaviour, and Poverty. In: Journal of Scottish Historical Studies 26 (2006), pp. 100–120.

Sturdy, Steve; Cooter, Roger: Science, Scientific Management, and the Transformation of Medicine in Britain, c. 1870–1950. In: History of Science 36 (1998), pp. 421–467.

Swift, Sarah H.: Training in Psychiatric Social Work at the Institute for Child Guidance 1927–1933. New York 1934.

Thomson, Mathew: Mental Hygiene as an International Movement. In: Weindling, Paul (ed.): International Health Organisations and Movements. Cambridge 1995, pp. 283–304.

Thomson, Mathew: Psychological Subjects: Identity, Culture, and Health in Twentieth Century Britain. Oxford 2006.

Timms, Noel: Psychiatric Social Work in Britain (1939–1962). London 1964.

Timms, Noel: Taking Social Work Seriously: the Contribution of the Functional School. In: British Journal of Social Work 27 (1997), pp. 723–737.

Turmel, André: A Historical Sociology of Childhood. Cambridge 2008.

Welshman, John: Evacuation and Social Policy during the Second World War: Myth and Reality. In: Twentieth Century British History 9 (1998), pp. 28–53.

Witmer, Helen Leland: By Way of Introduction. In: Smith College Studies in Social Work 1 (1930), pp. 1–5.

Wolf, Katherine M.: Evacuation of Children in Wartime: A Survey of the Literature, with Bibliography. In: The Psychoanalytic Study of the Child 1 (1945), pp. 389–404.

Socratic stories as vehicles of health education. The case of Johann Jakob Gabriel's "Von den Mitteln die Gesundheit zu erhalten"

Andreas Golob

Introduction

First published in 1792 and surviving in its second edition of 1802, Johann Jakob Gabriel's compilation "On the Means to Preserve Health"[1] represents one of the earliest attempts[2] to replace monotonous instructions like Bernhard Christoph Faust's "Catechism of Health". Its compiler, a humble Styrian priest and catechist, may be understood as a representative of the enlightened clergy who had internalised the reforms of the 1780s. Beyond his service as a pastor at relatively wealthy locations, he used his spare time to compile pedagogical books.[3]

---

1 Gabriel (1802). The first edition is only evident in a newspaper advertisement, cf. Zaunrith (1792).
2 Cf. the bibliography in Stroß (2000), p. 360.
3 Gabriel (1800); Gabriel (1802); Gabriel (1803) – he obviously plagiarised Friedrich Eberhard von Rochow's same-titled book of 1786, cf. also Gabriel (1795). It is possible to trace Gabriel's life (1758–1841) in Diözesanarchiv Graz (hereafter DAG), Personalakte Johann Jakob Gabriel. Especially his request to obtain a higher pension as a deficient priest, filed on February 25, 1836, reveals authentic and intimate details of his curriculum vitae. After completing five years of theological instructions, which the student had partly financed by private tutoring, and having served as "prefect of fifth year students of theology" he finished his education at the newly established General Seminar and was ordained as a priest in 1784. His career started in 1786 in the market town of Wildon where the young priest not only served as second chaplain and as catechist but also as second teacher (because the schoolmaster had been suspended). Four years later he continued his twofold duties in Hartberg; among others the cleric taught the second and third forms at the local school, and stayed there for eight years. The rest of his professional life – except for an interruption from 1804 to 1807 when he administrated the prestigious church district of Straßgang near Graz – was spent at the rural community of Feldkirchen where he supported the elderly parish priest. Officially pensioned in 1815 (as the certificate, issued on March 1, 1815, testifies) he still rendered auxiliary services in Graz and in particular in Feldkirchen until the early 1830s. Gabriel died at the Hospital of the Brothers of St. John of God in Graz where he had been accepted in 1832 and had assisted at the religious services for as long as he was able to carry out his duties. Furthermore Gabriel can be found in the records of Graz University when he entered the adjoined grammar school in 1770, see Universitätsbibliothek Graz, Abteilung für Sondersammlungen (hereafter UBG Sosa), Hs. 58, Vol. 1, 1770, Ex Parva. According to the entry in the baptismal registers of the Graz parish church 'Zum heiligen Blut' his father Mathias was a middle-class master craftsman, cf. DAG, Taufmatriken, Stadtpfarre Graz, July 24, 1758. Unfortunately no school visitation protocols from Gabriel's time in Wildon and Hartberg have survived. Cf. also Winklern (1810), pp. 46–47, for a short biographical valuation. On the General

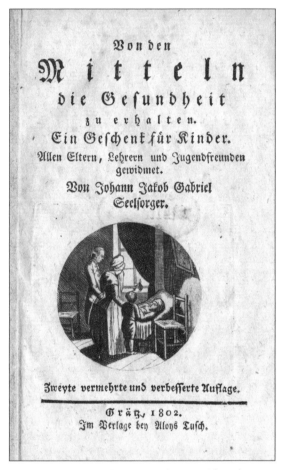

Figure 1: Title page of Johann Jakob Gabriel's health manual (1802)

The article itself is divided into three parts. The first one will provide the background and focus on medical law and canon law. Manuals of the 1790s will be considered to illustrate how the clergy responded to the regulations in theory and practice.[4] Newspaper articles and advertisements can show public expectations. The second part will introduce Gabriel's collection and highlight

Seminar that was founded to reform clerical education along Joseph II's ideas: Schöff-mann (1974). For an overview of the Styrian school system in the era of enlightened re-forms: Pietsch (1977).

4   Peck (1797); Poiger: Epistel (1791); Poiger: Kirchspiele (1791); Poiger: Häuserbesuche (1791). On the subject of "pastoral medicine" in general: Pompey (1968), pp. 74–289. Concerning religious as well as secular clergy in France: Delaunay (1948), pp. 84–110 and 118–135. More recently Kuhn (2003), pp. 211–221. On priests as agents of the health ad-ministration in Lower Austria in the late eighteenth and early nineteenth centuries espe-cially Weißensteiner (1997). Cf. for clerical combatants against smallpox (which was, however, neglected in Gabriel's compilation): Pammer (1995), pp. 21–29.

stylistic as well as thematic characteristics. Concluding remarks will dwell on opportunities of spreading the book and its contents.

Clergy and health system

By the 1780s, the expertise of accredited medical practitioners generally dominated over the priests' position at first glance. Funerals without official certificates of death were outlawed[5], and cemeteries had to meet adequate health standards[6]. Moreover, medical doctors were no longer obliged to take solemn oaths at their graduation ceremony.[7] On the other hand, the absolutist legislator compelled physicians to contact priests when their patients did not show any signs of recovery after the third visit.[8] If the sick refused extreme unction, medical treatment would even have to be stopped.[9] Midwives were instructed to baptise endangered newborns, even including minute details on how to consecrate conjoined twins.[10] Both regulations underlined the vital importance of traditional sacraments.

Furthermore, priests exercised administrative functions. Above all, the parish priests kept the baptismal, matrimonial and burial registers[11] which served as primary indicators in observing the outcomes of population politics. The clergy was supposed to participate actively in these efforts by preventing marriages between mentally or physically disabled prospective spouses.[12] Priests also testified the poverty of pregnant women, who should be admitted to state care[13], and also accredited and paid communal foster mothers[14]. Finally, the clergy was integrated in the warning system against cattle plagues.

---

5   Iohn (1790–1798), vol. I, pp. 164–178, vol. V, p. 205, vol. VI, pp. 423, 459 and 475. The collection offers an overview of the instructions implemented until the 1790s. Most of them originated in the eighteenth century and especially during the reigns of both Maria Theresia (1740–1780) and Joseph II (1780–1790). Cf. the chronological list at the end of Iohn (1790–1798), vol. IV: for laws before the seventeenth century pp. 3–7, for the seventeenth century pp. 7–12, for the eighteenth century pp. 12–120, for the period between 1740 and 1780 pp. 20–74. In his systematic summary, the author did not forget to include a short special category which dealt with ecclesiastical matters: Iohn (1790–1798), vol. IV, pp. 54–56. This aspect contained entries on abortion, sacraments and particularly baptism, funerals, oaths and epidemic diseases. Of course the regulations must still be judged against the opportunities of implementation, cf. Schlumbohm (1997), especially pp. 651 and 663 (concerning schools).
6   On these reforms in Styria: Payer (2003).
7   Iohn (1790–1798), vol. I, p. 264.
8   Iohn (1790–1798), vol. II, p. 163. According to Mezler (1808), p. 208, this law originated from a papal edict of 1566.
9   Iohn (1790–1798), vol. III, p. 359.
10 Iohn (1790–1798), vol. II, pp. 305–309.
11 Iohn (1790–1798), vol. II, pp. 240–243.
12 Iohn (1790–1798), vol. I, p. 258, and vol. II, p. 40.
13 Iohn (1790–1798), vol. I, p. 346.
14 Iohn (1790–1798), vol. I, p. 355.

Specific advice should be spread by reading out instructions from Johann Gottlieb Wollstein's manual when cattle plagues threatened the parish. Due to their close contact with the populace, clerics were considered to be the first to be informed in case of suspicious signs.[15]

The clergy was also instructed to teach and socially control the parish communities. The campaign against abortion, for instance, showed remorseless traits, because it stressed strict dogmatic positions. According to the official clerical standpoint, preachers and confessors should refute the popular notion that foetuses could not be condemned to hell.[16] On the other hand, the spirit of Enlightenment served as motivation when clerics were ordered to help to dispose of the prejudice that suicide victims should not be touched. In this context, the duty to administer first aid in any case was affirmed.[17] Last but not least, superstitious practices were to be condemned in general. The consecration of herbs[18] was deemed to be useless, and amulets[19] were strictly forbidden. The ringing of bells during thunderstorms[20] was banned for security reasons. A last announcement recommended that secular as well as clerical authorities should study Adalbert Vinzenz Zarda's handbook to familiarize themselves with the current standard of medical practices for non-professionals.[21]

The cited regulations could also be found in Schwerdling's compendium[22] which approached the question from the ecclesiastical point of view. In addition, it offered insights into how far non-theological matters constituted a part of the ecclesiastical education. Especially the "General Seminaries"[23] of the Josephinist decade focused – for instance – on natural history or agriculture. As far as teaching methods were concerned, prospective pastors learned the same techniques as secular primary school teachers. The entry on "preachers"[24] revealed the central duty of transmitting the gathered enlightened knowledge to the parish communities. The "practical teachings of Christianity" claimed priority and became joined not only to "virtue" but also to "Enlightenment" and "reason". Furthermore, the enlightened parish priest heralded edicts of all kinds to introduce and enforce the Sovereign's legislation.

---

15 Iohn (1790–1798), vol. V, p. 115.
16 Iohn (1790–1798), vol. I, pp. 4–5.
17 Iohn (1790–1798), vol. VI, p. 405.
18 Iohn (1790–1798), vol. II, p. 161.
19 Iohn (1790–1798), vol. V, p. 9.
20 Iohn (1790–1798), vol. VI, p. 574–575.
21 Iohn (1790–1798), vol. VI, p. 559. Note Zarda's ambition to especially educate parsons in rural areas: Siegert (2001).
22 E. g. on funerals: Schwerdling (1790), pp. 71–73 and 222–223. On certificates of poverty: pp. 157 and 165. On ringing the bells in thunderstorms: pp. 233–234. On registers: pp. 352–358.
23 Schwerdling (1790), pp. 177–182.
24 Schwerdling (1790), pp. 276–281.

Beyond sermonising, the clergy's role as part of the school authorities was crucial.[25] Religious education at primary school level became more closely linked to spreading general elementary knowledge, too. For instance, a companion to catechism included an example of a lesson on thunderstorms.[26] The anonymous author only dedicated the last two pages to praise the majestic nature of the phenomenon which should inspire veneration, but in non-superstitious ways. The rest of the sixteen page lesson dwelled on physical details as well as negative and especially positive effects. Neither did the clerical teacher forget to promote mandatory security arrangements and unmask useless practices. Last but not least, he tried to convince his listeners to install innovative lightning protectors which had been scientifically approved. Of course, he also explained in detail how they worked. With regard to medically induced laws in this field, the instruction that girls were not allowed to wear corsets in school could be quoted.[27]

The most common contact between clergy and accredited healers occurred when both carried out their duties at the sick bed. Burghard Peck's guide for inexperienced pastors discussed their relationship already in the introductory notes.[28] According to him, physicians often avoided consulting priests because they assumed that patients might fear that they soon had to die. The author attributed this argument to bad experiences with poorly trained priests. However, he also replied that physicians who acted this way not only sinned, but also defied the above cited laws. In his opinion, physicians and priests should ideally support each other by encouraging confidence in both professions, and he insisted that health had to be restored physically as well as spiritually. The competencies had to be sharply separated, though. Whereas medical treatment cared for the body, the priest cured the soul and was literally referred to as "doctor of the soul". Illness was in this case still traditionally linked to the patients' sinful behaviour or to a certain kind of divine purpose and should principally be met with catharsis and patience. Although priests would normally avoid interfering in physical cures, Peck recommended comprehensive knowledge, especially when patients approached the end of their lives. Thus, he listed no less than sixteen physical, emotional and social signs for this state and warned his colleagues that patients could remain in a condition of apparent death for a long time.[29] His illustrating examples were drawn from medical experts like Johann August Unzer, Johann Peter Frank and even Ambroise Paré to name only the most prominent. For example, the

25 Schwerdling (1790), pp. 293–302.
26 N.N. (1796). Cf. for the concept as such: Irminger (1788), pp. [III–XIV].
27 Schwerdling (1790), p. 237.
28 Peck (1797), pp. [III–XI]. From the physicians' perspective particularly Mezler (1808) who cited positive (pp. 125–126, 139–140, 201–202, 216) as well as negative (pp. 102, 117) practical examples of clerical interventions and testified concrete personal contacts between the two professions (pp. 102, 191–192).
29 Peck (1797), pp. 28–33. Cf. Mezler's criticism and his more comprehensive approach: Mezler (1808), pp. 214–221.

ideal pastor knew that fainting could ease the patients' suffering, as patients who recovered after serious illnesses had witnessed, or that spasms were natural phenomena, and he would console present relatives by referring to these facts.[30] In order to protect their own lives, priests had to be familiar with methods of avoiding infection. For this purpose, the manual included medically approved prescriptions and offered guidelines for adequate conduct at the sick bed, but also dietetic tips for a healthy life in general.[31] Peck only casually mentioned that, apart from their professional duties, clerics should use their knowledge as <u>philanthropists</u> to provide help in emergencies.[32] In this context, elementary information on prevention was also briefly brought up. Regarding details, Peck finally advised his readers to confront drunkards, who were not seriously ill, with the physical, mental and social outcomes of their sinful intemperance.[33] Further general admonitions against alcohol and opulent eating habits were obviously aimed at preventing addiction.

Benedikt Poiger exceeded this traditional framework most decidedly. In his magazine, he advocated that priests should act as active intermediaries between patients and physicians in scarcely developed regions. The clerical part would include reports for the doctors who could prescribe more appropriate treatments on this basis.[34] For emergencies, the parish priest should maintain a "private pharmacy", which did not actually conform to official regulations, in order to prolong the first, comparably harmless stage of diseases until a physician would become available. Furthermore, the clergy was not only entitled to prosecute charlatans but even to admonish incompetent barber surgeons. Poiger's examples also show that there were indeed priests who engaged in health education. One of his colleagues in Salzburg – at that time not part of the Habsburg Monarchy – did not limit his private Sunday and holiday lectures to the New Testament. Additionally, he recited instructions on first aid for casualties who had nearly drowned and suffocated or were struck by lightning. He also read out passages of Adam Andreas Senfft's catechism of health and of Joseph Weber's booklet on preventive measures in thunderstorms.[35] Another parish priest considered health issues when he exercised his regular and formal visits to the households in his community.[36] Two of the protocols revealed, among other details, consecrated means applied to alleviate diseases, superstitious formulae and the presence of popular herbal medicine.

30   Peck (1797), p. 27.
31   Peck (1797), pp. 172–184.
32   Peck (1797), p. 11.
33   Peck (1797), pp. 120–126.
34   Poiger: Epistel (1791), p. 12. For the following remarks: pp. 13–14. The idea probably came from Heinrich Gottlieb Zerrenner's "Volksbuch", cf. Poiger: Gemein-Bibliothek (1791), pp. 66–67.
35   Poiger: Epistel (1791), pp. 26–27.
36   Poiger: Häuserbesuche (1791).

Public opinion generally reflected the priests' estimation and goals. Similar expectations can be traced in the *Bauernzeitung* ("Peasants' Newspaper") which was not only widely distributed in rural areas – as the name would suggest – but also in Styrian towns. In 1792, the educational, multidisciplinary supplements contained a contribution which discussed positive and negative effects of visits on the recovery of patients.[37] The anonymous author demanded that "sensible" priests should approach sick and dying people in a strictly unobtrusive way. Not only for lay visitors but also for the clergy, the patient's bedroom was to be seen as a "sanctuary". One year earlier, Klaudius Martin Scherer, a Tyrolean physician, who himself edited a weekly popular periodical on health care, shared one of his cases which featured an "upright priest" who advised a woman to use herbal drugs under medical supervision instead of seeking solely religious cures against an alleged bedevilment.[38] According to book advertisements, priests ranked among the enlightened propagators of pedagogical literature. Like school inspectors, landlords and philanthropists, they could profit from discounts.[39] Especially catechists were invited to distribute books as presents after successful examinations. Lists of such prizes included the most recommendable pedagogical titles. One of them also included an up-to-date Viennese version of Faust's "Catechism of Health".[40]

Gabriel's collection of Socratic stories

Since Gabriel did not invent the stories himself[41], they may demonstrate routes of cultural transfer. No less than nine of the 27 stories can be traced to Rochow's "Kinderfreund", a groundbreaking reader of the mid-1770s.[42] Another narrative was first published in Peter Villaume's manual for teachers.[43] On the

37 N.N. (1792), p. 505.
38 Scheerer [sic] (1791).
39 The local bookseller Johann Andreas Kienreich, for instance, sold a copy of Friedrich Eberhard von Rochow's prominent reader "Der Kinderfreund" at roughly three quarters of the normal price when the customer took at least a dozen: Kienreich (1795). Johann Joseph Mayr's bookshop, situated in Salzburg and represented by Kienreich, Franz Ferstl and Alois Tusch in Graz, even conceded forty percent off on literary works of Ägidius Jais, a Benedictine monk who was a leading proponent of the campaign against masturbation in the Southern German countries, cf. Mayr (1796). On Jais' crusade see e. g. Bloch (1998), pp. 497–518.
40 Kienreich (1797).
41 Rudolph Zacharias Becker overtly recommended that teachers should compile personal collections. Cf. Völpel (1996), p. 153.
42 The pages in brackets refer to Gabriel (1802). Rochow (1776), nos. 28 (pp. 52–53), 32 (pp. 54–55), 53 (p. 57), 54 (p. 59), 60 (pp. 73–74), 71 (pp. 44–45), and Rochow (1779), nos. 27 (pp. 53–54), 39 (pp. 39–41), 40 (pp. 59–60). See for Rochow: Schmitt (2001); Völpel (1996), pp. 59–106; for his influence on Habsburg-ruled Hungary especially Németh (2007).
43 Villaume (1787), p. 90 (pp. 13–14). (Villaume, a Huguenot, held a position as preacher in Halberstadt.)

basis of these pieces of evidence, the influence of Prussian-ruled territories is conspicuous. A further five stories from Rudolph Zacharias Becker's "Noth- und Hülfs-Büchlein"[44] and no less than eight narratives from Christian Gotthilf Salzmann's "Elementarbuch"[45] prove the importance of the Central German countries. The preface also mentioned Faust's "Catechism of Health", though only to criticise its monotonous style.[46] On the other hand, the collection was well received in Salzburg.[47]

The lively narratives allow various approaches to interpretation. Young-sters were addressed in a personal way. Apart from the 25 fictional stories and two dialogues, practical instructions which primarily focused on accidents such as the apparent death from cold, drowning or suffocating, as well as sen-sible explanations tried to convince the young audience. The ideal way to preserve health was seen in the "habit" of observing a modest lifestyle. The very first example illustrated examples of dietetically wise behaviour.[48] "Mis-ter Oront" taught his obedient children to prefer vegetables and fruit to meat. Sweets were not allowed. Moreover, the father avoided overheating his off-spring's rooms and beds. The children also had to endure cold weather, and fresh water served to harden and clean their bodies. This treatment resulted in their physically visible well-being which was expressed by metaphors of na-ture such as "juvenile glow", rosy-red cheeks and energetic "young deer".[49] In contrast, "Herr Weichlich", that is "Mister Weak", spoiled his four children who became sickly and were drastically as well as realistically described as "miserable" figures with "yellow" skin, "blue lips", "shrunken eyes", decayed teeth and a generally weak constitution. At a dinner at Mister Oront's house

---

44 Becker (1789), pp. 92–93 (pp. 21–22), p. 93 (p. 22), p. 100 (pp. 23–24), pp. 114–115 (pp. 19–20), p. 115 (pp. 20–21). On Becker: Völpel (1996), pp. 129–186.

45 Salzmann (1787), pp. 1–6 (pp. 5–10), pp. 6–7 (pp. 27–28) – taken from [Joachim Heinrich] Campe, p. 47 (pp. 30–31), pp. 50–51 (pp. 32–33), pp. 51–52 (pp. 17–18) – signed [Johann Georg] Sulzer, p. 52 (p. 18), pp. 56–58 (pp. 25–26), pp. 59–60 (pp. 16–17) – originally in "Goldner Spiegel". Cf. for Salzmann in general Völpel (1996), pp. 187–189. On the "Ele-mentarbuch": Brunken (1982).

46 Gabriel (1802), p. 4. Cf. for this criticism in particular Böning (1990), pp. 39–40. On liter-ary forms as alternatives, with an overview concerning health issues: Alzheimer-Haller (2004), pp. 280–331. See for general tendencies in the Habsburg monarchy (though very short and incomplete on Styria) Seibert (1987), pp. 107–108. Last but not least on the in-teresting interdependencies between narratives or case stories on the one hand and self-perceptions as well as articulations of personal life stories on the other: Stolberg (2003), pp. 66–68 and 271–277.

47 N.N.: Von den Mitteln die Gesundheit zu erhalten (1793). NB that Gabriel's efforts were rewarded by accredited physicians who normally fought against non-professional utter-ances under the leadership of the journal's editors Johann Jakob Hartenkeil and Franz Xaver Mezler. Even Faust's approach went too far due to its comprehensive and there-fore counterproductive contents, cf. N.N.: Entwurf zu einem Gesundheitskatechismus (1793).

48 Gabriel (1802), pp. 5–6.

49 Gabriel (1802), p. 7.

they were not able to enjoy their meals.[50] However, as the most horrifying outcome, three of the children died at an early age. Two siblings succumbed to ordinary colds after playing outside in winter.[51] No less than sixteen of the 27 episodes had fatal endings.[52] This ultimate form of deterrent should not just be dismissed as a negative and repulsive method of education.[53] It must also be interpreted against the background of high rates of infant mortality, threats of epidemic diseases and scarce health care facilities. On the other hand, the first, longest and thus probably most prominent story also highlighted the evils of supersaturated societies.

Whereas physical motives dominated at the beginning, mental, social and, last but not least, religious aspects had their share, too. For instance, fear exacerbated the impact of a thunderstorm[54], and a superstitious young man, who mistook a chimney sweeper for a ghost at a nocturnal encounter, nearly died of a cold which he contracted when running away[55]. The latter case additionally displayed social reactions by mentioning that old people as well as young children ridiculed the unfortunate fellow. A naïve young boy, who neglected personal hygiene when his kind-hearted but busy parents were not present, was shunned by decent society because of his bad breath and his yellowish body covered with "rash" and "vermin".[56] With regard to supporting facets of society, rudimentary first aid measures were deemed to be compulsory.[57] Only one story portrayed donations to a disabled beggar who was himself responsible for his handicap.[58] Given the main thrust of the stories, that everyone was held accountable for his or her own health, this marginal appearance does not surprise. Lastly, a highly responsible servant, who lay terminally ill after his master's mad dog had bitten him, wanted to be tied, in order not to hurt anyone in his agony.[59]

A young adult's fate[60] could exemplarily link social and religious contexts[61]. Addicted to sweets since his early childhood[62], when he had been se-

---

50 Gabriel (1802), pp. 6–7.
51 Gabriel (1802), p. 9.
52 Gabriel (1802), pp. 5–10, 13–14, 16–17, 19–20, 20–21, 22, 23–24, 27–28, 39–41, 48–49, 51–52, 52–53, 53–54, 59, 59–60, 73–74. Cf. Nassen (1988), p. 68.
53 Note that Walter Benjamin preferred this uncompromising, drastic and honest style to glossed over and childish tendencies at the beginning of the 20th century, cf. Benjamin (1969), pp. 42–44.
54 Gabriel (1802), pp. 44–45.
55 Gabriel (1802), pp. 54–55.
56 Gabriel (1802), pp. 32–33.
57 Gabriel (1802), p. 66 (in general deliberations).
58 Gabriel (1802), pp. 46–47.
59 Gabriel (1802), pp. 48–49.
60 Gabriel (1802), pp. 16–17.
61 According to Völpel (1996), pp. 73–74, 88–89, 93, 99 and, respectively, 166–168, Rochow as well as Becker quoted biblical texts such as parts of the New Testament or proverbs of Solomon and Jesus Sirach in order to enhance the acceptance of their story collections.
62 It is intriguing that Gabriel listed "figs, almonds, apples and pears", whereas his precursors originally talked of "raisins, almonds and confection".

duced by his wet nurse[63], he squandered all the money that his parents had sent him. At last, he even stole money from his employer sliding – so to say – into drug-related crime. In order to evade fair secular justice for his shameful behaviour, the miscreant signed on a ship to escape to East India. On his way, "divine" revenge struck, and he perished when the ship capsized. On the other hand, a virtuous and devout lifestyle helped to face deadly illnesses[64], and religious exercises were especially recommended for diseases of the soul such as "melancholy"[65]. Further examples of misconduct could be interpreted in terms of the seven cardinal sins. A stereotypically greedy Jew died during an epidemic because he wanted to draw profit from an infected ox skin.[66] An envious peasant woman died of "bilious fever" when her neighbour inherited a substantial amount of money.[67] Another protagonist killed a child, who had injured one of his infant relatives, in wrath and was sentenced to death.[68] Gluttony was of course prominent in the six stories which dealt with harmful eating[69] and/or drinking habits, including alcohol[70] abuse.

The inexpressive and cautious contribution on lust[71], which did not explicitly name the committed sins, leads over to those three stories which involved priests. Most likely, the young sinner, who received his extreme unction in an infirmary, was guilty of extramarital sexual intercourse and had been infected with an unspecified venereal disease.[72] The doomed, remorseful patient wished he had been warned of "debauchery" earlier in his life. The decent priest consoled his client and confirmed his findings. In a second example a pastor's admonition was of no avail.[73] Little Klaus, suffering from itching eczema, did not obey his "sensible cleric", who ordered him not to scratch, and he had to die as a consequence. The last relevant episode featured a parish priest who was confronted with an epidemic disease.[74] His parishioners were split over how to tackle the situation. Some families trusted in the shepherd's traditional healing know-how and had to bemoan a high death rate.

---

63 For the debate on wet nurses Toppe (1993), pp. 119–189.

64 Gabriel (1802), pp. 73–74.

65 Gabriel (1802), pp. 55–56 (in general comments). Cf. for growing caution concerning mental diseases: Roth (1979), pp. 314–318.

66 Gabriel (1802), pp. 20–21.

67 Gabriel (1802), pp. 52–53.

68 Gabriel (1802), pp. 53–54. NB that this episode and the preceding one were taken from Friedrich Eberhard von Rochow who did not centre on health issues in these stories.

69 Gabriel (1802), pp. 5–10, 13–14, 14–15, 16–17, 18.

70 Gabriel (1802), pp. 14–15, 25–26. Cf. Stach (2002), p. 198.

71 Gabriel (1802), pp. 51–52.

72 Note that masturbation also ranked prominently in the context of unchastity. For instance, Peck's position regarding unchaste behaviour proved to be rather relentless. Especially masturbation, as previously described by the physician Simon André Tissot, would degrade addicted persons to a state "below the unreasoning animal". By the way, the same was true of homosexual practices which were alluded to in the following paragraph. Cf. Peck (1797), pp. 111–112.

73 Gabriel (1802), p. 59.

74 Gabriel (1802), pp. 39–41.

Others relied on the clergyman's expertise on up-to-date fundamental health care knowledge and obediently consulted a licensed physician, as they were told. Hence, most of them were spared. On the whole, these stories thus echoed contemporary views on clerical visits to sick community members and the enlightened clergy's role as an educated and authoritative part of the social elite.

Starting from the last example, various agents of health care and propagators of knowledge can finally be identified. Principally, licensed healers represented the first choice for Gabriel.[75] However, the catechist also felt obliged to rebut popular prejudices against avaricious licensed physicians[76], thereby revealing obstacles to his ideal. If physicians were not available, educated, enlightened role models would come to the fore. Apart from priests, well educated friends[77] could be traced, and in the closing story[78], schools were praised, too. Within the families, responsible parents[79], particularly fathers[80], and older, more experienced siblings[81] did their share. In the latter cases, two sisters warned their younger brothers. Male children normally ranked among the imprudent, disobedient characters who had to learn their lesson the hard way. On the other hand, "wise men, aged mothers, executioners, marketers"[82], wet nurses and shepherds played malicious counterparts.

Reception and concluding remarks

To conclude, enlightened positions encouraged the Catholic clergy to participate more actively in the physical health system of the Habsburg Monarchy in the second half of the eighteenth century. Theoretical and practical examples of intensified clerical education and leadership in health issues as well as in other, non-theological contexts could, moreover, suggest that the priests were in some sense actually upgraded to serve as important members of the absolutist state, and not downgraded to mere bureaucrats in an increasingly secular and rational environment. True, the clergy was subjugated to the control of li-

---

75 Gabriel (1802), pp. 13–14, 19–20, 21–22, 23–24, 27–28, 39–41, 57 (a "sensible" [!] "barber surgeon"), 59–60. After accidents, the author also recommended to seek professional help as soon as possible, cf. Gabriel (1802), pp. 66–71.

76 Gabriel (1802), pp. 57–58.

77 Gabriel (1802), pp. 30–31, 44–45.

78 Gabriel (1802), pp. 73–74.

79 Gabriel (1802), pp. 21–22, 59–60, 73–74.

80 Gabriel (1802), pp. 5–10, 46–47. Cf. Wild (1987), pp. 205–257. On mothers as healers recently Ritzmann (2008), pp. 87–91.

81 Gabriel (1802), pp. 14–15, 16–17. NB that female household members were generally in charge of health issues. Given the extraordinary importance of nutrition, they were key figures in health maintenance. All in all, Gabriel actually neglected this connection.

82 Gabriel (1802), p. 50 (in general remarks). See the stories above for the last two professions. For the Styrian situation in the eighteenth and nineteenth centuries cf. Hammer-Luza (2005).

censed physicians, but both were answerable to governmental authorities and obliged to maintain a friendly coexistence. Clerical responsibilities and know-how concerning health were also suitable to enhance the public esteem of the priests which itself requested and influenced these services to a certain extent. The importance of the sacraments of baptism and extreme unction remained unaffected. Lay professionals such as physicians and midwives were even officially ordered to recommend or administer these ceremonies. Attempts to abandon superstitious customs certainly purified the church but did not necessarily lead to more secular approaches. The absolutist regime did not even shy away from using traditional dogmata when they seemed appropriate to achieve official aims and to maintain social discipline. In the case of mental illness, clerical cure and explanations were still accepted.

Within this framework, Johann Jakob Gabriel was extraordinarily active as an eloquent propagator of health knowledge. Although the stories were not his brainchildren, his efforts in compiling a whole collection of them and supplying them with general comments must not be underestimated. His occupation as an enlightened catechist offered opportunities to lecture not only on dogmata but also on practical know-how such as preventive health care. Since lack of education was seen as a major obstacle to the prevention of disease, his popular and vivid approach must have been regarded as an ideal way to improve public health. The author himself seems to have been quite conscious of his achievements. When he filed his first plea for pension on March 25, 1803[83], he pointed out his remarkable efforts in schools and as an educator of the youth in general. Moreover, his second (and successful) attempt was, among others, explicitly recommended by the clerical authorities on December 28, 1814 due to his "composition of several much-lauded educational writings".[84] It is also evident that the collection "Von den Mitteln die Gesundheit zu erhalten" was distributed as a present to pupils with distinguished examination

---

83 DAG, Personalakte Johann Jakob Gabriel.
84 DAG, Personalakte Johann Jakob Gabriel. It might be of interest that Gabriel repeatedly hinted at his bad physical constitution. His second request of November 30, 1814 revealed that he had developed severe inguinal hernia as early as 1803, and more recently he had suffered from scrotal hernia which caused spasms over two or more hours even after moderate meals. When he asked for a higher pension on February 25, 1836, Gabriel also noted that he had taken a short time out after his exhausting studies (that had been accompanied by additional duties, see above), following the advice of physicians. These details apparently set the personal background for Gabriel's zeal to teach youngsters how to become and remain healthy.

results.[85] Finally the preface[86] to his "Denksprüche", that he signed as "teacher and friend", sheds some light on Gabriel's teaching methods. Each week, the teacher used to write one of the aphorisms on the blackboard and tell a story on the specific subject. Gabriel also recalled that his listeners, who were directly addressed as recipients in the prologue, followed his narratives in "silent attention". After their time at school, the busy former pupils should memorise one aphorism of the book a week and at the same time remember the fictional example. Surprisingly, Gabriel did not mention (Socratic) questions in this context, although they had become fundamental to secular as well as religious instructions by the end of the eighteenth century. In Styria, for instance, an "instruction for catechists", which circulated in 1806, officially endorsed Socrates' method and related it to Jesus Christ's approach. The catechists were instructed to analyse their educational material and to separate it into suitable divisions and subdivisions. Then they should teach in the "most informal, friendly and entertaining way". As an ideal outcome, one targeted question after the other would lead the thoughtful and attentive pupils to intellectual findings "as if they had found everything themselves". The teaching style should aim at the children's senses and include as many narratives as possible.[87]

Of course, it is hard to actually assess the impact of Gabriel's lessons. When Victor Fossel, the first historian of medicine at Graz University, conducted ethnographic field research in Styria at the end of the nineteenth cen-

85 Cf. the list in Steiermärkisches Landesarchiv, Gubernium (Gub.), Fasz. 74 – 1806, 6977: Verzeichniß Jener Bücher, welche bisher [until 1806] bey öffentlichen Prüfungen in dieser Diözes [Graz-Seckau] vertheilet worden sind. The overview – briefly and superficially discussed in Pietsch (1977), pp. 137–138 – encompasses 92 books which were given away in the administrative districts of Graz and Maribor. Gabriel's three books can be identified and were awarded to successful pupils in and around Graz. The report for Maribor (Marburg an der Drau) probably only refers to his "Denksprüche". Cf. also the subtitles of Gabriel (1802): "A present for children. Dedicated to all parents, teachers and friends of young people".

86 Gabriel (1800), Vorrede. Whereas his compilation on the means to preserve health was "only" reprinted once, this book achieved its fourth edition in 1815 which could rudimentarily prove extraordinary public demand and/or distribution rates. By the way, one copy that found its way into the New York Public Library conquered the World Wide Web: http://books.google.at/books?id=4k0CAAAAYAAJ&printsec=front cover&dq=%22joha nn+jakob+gabriel%22#v=onepage&q=&f=false (last access: January 15, 2010). For local collections of aphorisms: Kunitsch (1797); Sperl (1817). On the interplay of proverbs on the one hand and narratives on the other: Völpel (1996), pp. 104 (on Rochow) and 169–172 (on Becker).

87 Steiermärkisches Landesarchiv, Gubernium (Gub.), Fasz. 74 – 1806, 2821: "Instruction für Katecheten". Note Kunitsch's anthology which explicitly referred to "Socratic" conversations: Kunitsch (1795). Cf. for Franz Michael Vierthaler's prominent deliberations on Socrates and their reflections in the education of catechists: Lentner (1955), pp. 203–218. See also pp. 108–111 for Franz Giftschütz whose guide on pastoral theology (first published in 1785) was recommended in the instruction. Cf. for Rochow's role as promoter of the Socratic method: Völpel (1996), p. 83.

tury[88], he still found a fair amount of superstitious practices and pre-Enlightenment knowledge that had obviously survived the enlightened campaigns. Scarce provisions of health care[89], which were only alluded to indirectly, and financial barriers to afford licensed medical advice and treatment, which were actually neglected in Gabriel's book, certainly also played their part in limiting his success.

Bibliography

Published Sources

Becker, Rudolph Zacharias: Noth- und Hülfs-Büchlein für Bauersleute oder lehrreiche Freuden- und Trauer-Geschichte des Dorfs Mildheim. Für Junge und Alte beschrieben. Graz 1789.

Gabriel, Johann Jakob: Wörter-Katechismus oder Erklärungen wichtiger Wörter nach ihren gemeinnützigsten Bedeutungen, und mit lehrreichen Beyspielen begleitet, für die Jugend. Graz 1795.

Gabriel, J[ohann] J[akob]: Denksprüche durch Beyspiele und Erzählungen erläutert für die Jugend. 2nd ed. Graz 1800.

Gabriel, Johann Jakob: Von den Mitteln die Gesundheit zu erhalten. Ein Geschenk für Kinder. Allen Eltern, Lehrern und Jugendfreunden gewidmet. 2nd, augmented and improved ed. Graz 1802.

Gabriel, Johann Jakob: Katechismus der gesunden Vernunft, oder Versuch in faßlichen Erklärungen wichtiger Wörter nach ihren gemeinnützigsten Bedeutungen, und mit einigen Beyspielen begleitet. Zur Beförderung richtiger und bessernder Erkenntniß für die Jugend. Graz 1803.

Iohn, Iohann Dionis: Lexikon der K. K. Medizinalgesetze. 6 vols. Prag 1790–1798.

[Irminger, Hans Ulrich:] Fragen an Kinder. Eine Einleitung zum Unterricht in der Religion. Von der Ascetischen Gesellschaft in Zürich. Wien 1788.

Kienreich, Joh[ann] Andreas: Bey Joh. Andreas Kienreich, Buch- und Musikalienhändler in Grätz, in der Herrengasse, im v. Frauenbergischen Hause, dem Rathhause gegenüber, ist ganz neu zu haben. In: Der Biedermann (December 23, 1795) [unpaginated].

Kienreich, Johann Andreas: Bücher, welche zu Prämien bey den Prüfungen gebraucht werden können. In: Grätzer Zeitung (August 14, 1797) [unpaginated].

Kunitsch, Michael: Versuch Sokratischer Gespräche über die Erzählungen in dem zweyten Theile des Lesebuches für Landschulen der k. k. Staaten. Graz 1795.

Kunitsch, Michael: Drey hundert fünfzig Sätze lehrreichen Inhaltes zu Vorschriften und zum Dictiren. Zusammengetragen zum Behufe für öffentliche und Privatlehrer der Deutschen Jugend. Graz 1797.

Mayr, [Johann Joseph]: Bei Herrn Ferstl, Tusch, und Kienreich Buchhändlern in Gratz ist zu haben. In: Grätzer Bürgerzeitung (February 19, 1796), Grätzer Zeitung (February 23, 1796), Der Steyrische Biedermann (February 29, 1796) [unpaginated].

Mezler, Franz Xaver: Ueber den Einfluß der Heilkunst auf die practische Theologie. Ein Beytrag zur Pastoralmedicin. 3rd, augmented ed. Vol. 2. Ulm 1808.

N.N.: Uiber die Krankenbesuche. In: Bauernzeitung (November 19, 1792), pp. 504–505.

---

88   Fossel (1885), e.g. p. 13. For a more scientific and neutral approach: Grabner (1997).

89   Cf. for the Styrian setting: Wimmer (1991), pp. 70–77. More recently on Graz Huber-Reismann (2003) and on Leoben Huber-Reismann (2009).

N.N.: Bückeburg bey Althans: Entwurf zu einem Gesundheitskatechismus für die Kirchen und Schulen der Grafschaft Schaumburg-Lippe. Verbesserte und vermehrte Auflage. 1793. 64 Seit. in 8vo. (Pr. 50 Exemplare einen Rthlr.). In: Medicinisch-chirurgische Zeitung 4 (1793), no. 3, pp. 84–95.

N.N.: Grätz bey K. Zaunrith: Von den Mitteln die Gesundheit zu erhalten. Ein Geschenk für Kinder. Allen Eltern, Lehrern und Jugendfreunden gewidmet. 1792. 67 S. in 8vo. (Pr. 5 Gr.). In: Medicinisch-chirurgische Zeitung 4 (1793), no. 2, pp. 46–48.

N.N.: Katechetische Beyspiele. 12. Vom Gewitter. In: Der Seelsorger in der Schule: Oder Sammlung gewählter Abhandlungen zu einem zweckmäßigen Schul- und Religionsunterricht, mit praktischen Beyspielen begleitet. Vol. 2. (= Allgemeines Magazin für Prediger, Seelsorger und Katecheten 9) Wien 1796, pp. 330–345.

Peck, Burghard: Der Seelsorger am Krankenbette: Oder systematische Anleitung für Seelsorger zu einem zweckmäßigen Verfahren und Behandlung der Kranken. (= Allgemeines Magazin für Prediger, Seelsorger und Katecheten 11) Wien 1797.

Poiger, Benedikt: Epistel an die Seelsorger und Priester. Ein ziemlich langer, aber nothwendiger Prolog. In: Der Priesterfreund 1 (1791), pp. 1–63.

Poiger, Benedikt: Wie könnte in jedem Kirchspiele eine nüzliche Gemein-Bibliothek am leichtesten errichtet werden? In: Der Priesterfreund 1 (1791), pp. 64–92.

Poiger, Benedikt: Von pfärrlichen Häuserbesuchen. In: Der Priesterfreund 1 (1791), pp. 92–117.

Rochow, Friedrich Eberhard von: Der Kinderfreund. Ein Lesebuch zum Gebrauch in Landschulen. Vol. 1. Brandenburg; Leipzig 1776; Vol. 2. Brandenburg; Leipzig 1779.

Salzmann, Christian Gotthilf: Moralisches Elementarbuch. Vol. 2. Leipzig 1787.

Scheerer [sic], [Klaudius Martin]: Von Präservativmitteln. In: Grazer Bauernzeitung (August 1, 1791) [unpaginated].

Schwerdling, Johann: Alphabetisches Handlexikon aller k. k. Verordnungen in geistlichen Sachen, vom Antritte der Regierung weiland Marien Theresien bis ersten Jäner 1790. Wien 1790.

Sperl, Franz Xaver: Lehrreiche Stoffe zu Vorschriften und zum Dictiren. Auch als Lese- und Memorirbuch für Kinder zu gebrauchen. 2nd ed. Graz 1817.

Villaume, [Peter]: Praktisches Handbuch für Lehrer in Bürger- und Land-Schulen. Wien 1787.

Zaunrith, Kaspar: Von den Mitteln die Gesundheit zu erhalten. Ein Geschenk für Kinder. Allen Eltern, Lehrern und Jugendfreunden gewidmet. Mit 1 Titel-Vignet, wie trostlose Eltern ihren sterbenden Sohn beweinen. Kostet 15 kr. In: Bauernzeitung (May 24, 1792), pp. 122–123.

Literature

Alzheimer-Haller, Heidrun: Handbuch zur narrativen Volksaufklärung. Moralische Geschichten 1780–1848. Berlin; New York 2004.

Benjamin, Walter: Alte Kinderbücher. In: Benjamin, Walter: Über Kinder, Jugend und Erziehung. (= edition suhrkamp 391) Frankfurt/Main 1969, pp. 39–46.

Bloch, Karl Heinz: Die Bekämpfung der Jugendmasturbation im 18. Jahrhundert. Ursachen – Verlauf – Nachwirkungen. (= Studien zur Sexualpädagogik 11) Frankfurt/Main et al 1998.

Böning, Holger: Medizinische Volksaufklärung und Öffentlichkeit. Ein Beitrag zur Popularisierung aufklärerischen Gedankengutes und zur Entstehung einer Öffentlichkeit über Gesundheitsfragen. Mit einer Bibliographie medizinischer Volksschriften. In: Internationales Archiv für Sozialgeschichte der deutschen Literatur 15 (1990), no. 1, pp. 1–92.

Brunken, Otto: Christian Gotthilf Salzmann (1744–1811): Moralisches Elementarbuch. In: Brüggemann, Theodor; Ewers, Hans-Heino (eds.): Handbuch zur Kinder- und Jugendliteratur. Von 1750 bis 1800. Stuttgart 1982, cols. 574–593.

Delaunay, Paul: La médecine et l'église. Contribution à l'histoire de l'exercice médical par les clercs. Paris 1948.

Fossel, Victor: Volksmedicin und medicinischer Aberglaube in Steiermark. Ein Beitrag zur Landeskunde. Graz 1885.

Grabner, Elfriede: Krankheit und Heilen. Eine Kulturgeschichte der Volksmedizin in den Ostalpen. (= Mitteilungen des Instituts für Gegenwartsvolkskunde 16; Sitzungsberichte der Philosophisch-historischen Klasse der Österreichischen Akademie der Wissenschaften 457) 2nd, revised ed., supplemented with an introduction. Wien 1997.

Hammer-Luza, Elke: Kurpfuscher und Bauernärzte vor den Schranken des Gerichts. Aspekte der steirischen Volksmedizin im 18. und 19. Jahrhundert. In: Riegler, Josef (ed.): Bauern, Bürger, hohe Herren. (= Veröffentlichungen des Steiermärkischen Landesarchivs 34) Graz 2005, pp. 51–71.

Huber-Reismann, Elfriede Maria: Krankheit, Gesundheitswesen und Armenfürsorge. In: Brunner, Walter (ed.): Geschichte der Stadt Graz. Vol. 2: Wirtschaft – Gesellschaft – Alltag. Graz 2003, pp. 239–356.

Huber-Reismann, Elfriede Maria: Die Medizinische Versorgung der Stadt Leoben vom 13. bis zum 20. Jahrhundert. Eine sozialhistorische Quellenstudie als Beitrag zur Medizingeschichte sowie zur Steirischen Stadtgeschichtsforschung. Diss. Phil. Graz 2009.

Kuhn, Thomas K.: Religion und neuzeitliche Gesellschaft. Studien zum sozialen und diakonischen Handeln in Pietismus, Aufklärung und Erweckungsbewegung. (= Beiträge zur historischen Theologie 122) Tübingen 2003.

Lentner, Leopold: Katechetik und Religionsunterricht in Österreich. Vol. 1: Katechetik als Universitätsdisziplin in der Zeit der Aufklärung. (= Veröffentlichungen des Erzbischöflichen Amtes für Unterricht und Erziehung 5) Innsbruck; Wien; München 1955.

Nassen, Ulrich: Diätetische Grundsätze im Spiegel der Kinder- und Jugendliteratur um 1800. Skizzen. In: Sprache und Literatur in Wissenschaft und Unterricht 19 (1988), no. 2, pp. 68–74.

Németh, András: Die Philanthropismus- und Rochowrezeption in Ungarn. In: Schmitt, Hanno; Horlacher, Rebekka; Tröhler, Daniel (eds.): Pädagogische Volksaufklärung im 18. Jahrhundert im europäischen Kontext: Rochow und Pestalozzi im Vergleich. (= Neue Pestalozzi-Studien 10) Bern; Stuttgart; Wien 2007, pp. 198–216.

Pammer, Michael: Vom Beichtzettel zum Impfzeugnis. Beamte, Ärzte, Priester und die Einführung der Vaccination. In: Österreich in Geschichte und Literatur 39 (1995), no. 1, pp. 11–29.

Payer, Eva: "… wegen des großen üblen Geruchs …". Veränderungen des Begräbniskultes in der Steiermark durch die Verordnungen Maria Theresias und Josephs II. In: Blätter für Heimatkunde 77 (2003), pp. 118–126.

Pietsch, Walter: Die Theresianische Schulreform in der Steiermark (1775–1805). Graz 1977.

Pompey, Heinrich: Die Bedeutung der Medizin für die kirchliche Seelsorge im Selbstverständnis der sogenannten Pastoralmedizin. Eine bibliographisch-historische Untersuchung bis zur Mitte des 19. Jahrhunderts. (= Untersuchungen zur Theologie der Seelsorge 23) Freiburg/Brsg.; Basel; Wien 1968.

Ritzmann, Iris: Sorgenkinder. Kranke und behinderte Mädchen und Jungen im 18. Jahrhundert. Köln; Weimar; Wien 2008.

Roth, Gottfried: Pastoralmedizinische und arztethische Probleme im Rahmen der Entwicklung der Nervenheilkunde im Österreich des 18. Jahrhunderts. In: Kovács, Elisabeth (ed.): Katholische Aufklärung und Josephinismus. Wien 1979, pp. 310–322.

Schlumbohm, Jürgen: Gesetze, die nicht durchgesetzt werden – ein Strukturmerkmal des frühneuzeitlichen Staates? In: Geschichte und Gesellschaft 23 (1997), no. 4, pp. 647–663.

Schmitt, Hanno: Der sanfte Modernisierer Friedrich Eberhard von Rochow: Eine Neuinter-
pretation. In: Schmitt, Hanno; Tosch, Frank (eds.): Vernunft fürs Volk. Friedrich Eberhard
von Rochow 1734–1805 im Aufbruch Preußens. Berlin 2001, pp. 11–34.

Schöffmann, Wolfgang: Das Generalseminar in Graz. Dipl.-Arb. theol. Graz 1974.

Seibert, Ernst: Jugendliteratur im Übergang vom Josephinismus zur Restauration, mit einem
bibliographischen Anhang über die österreichische Kinder- und Jugendliteratur von 1770–
1830. (= Literatur und Leben, Neue Folge 38) Wien; Köln; Graz 1987.

Siegert, Reinhart: Zarda, Adalbert Vinzenz: Ist es zweckmäßig und zulässig, die angehenden
Landseelsorger in einer eingeschränkten Volksarzneykunde zu unterrichten? Bey Eröff-
nung der außerordentlich-öffentlichen Vorlesungen über die Rettungsmittel in Plötzlichen
Lebensgefahren im Jahre 1793 beantwortet von Adalbert Vinzenz Zarda. In: Siegert, Reinhart; Böning, Holger: Volksaufklärung. Biobibliographisches Handbuch zur Popularisierung aufklärerischen Denkens im deutschen Sprachraum von den Anfängen bis 1850.
Vol. 2.2: Der Höhepunkt der Volksaufklärung 1781–1800 und die Zäsur durch die Franzö-
sische Revolution. Stuttgart-Bad Cannstatt 2001, col. 1911.

Stach, Reinhard: Über Diebe, Dirnen, Süchtige und Waisen. Christian Gotthilf Salzmann und
die sozialen Randgruppen. In: Gutjahr, Elisabeth; Habel, Werner (eds.): Lebendige Tradition. Festschrift für Helmut Heiland. Hohengehren 2002, pp. 191–213.

Stolberg, Michael: Homo patiens. Krankheits- und Körpererfahrung in der Frühen Neuzeit.
Köln; Weimar; Wien 2003.

Stroß, Annette M[iriam]: Pädagogik und Medizin. Ihre Beziehungen in "Gesundheitserzie-
hung" und wissenschaftlicher Pädagogik 1779–1933. (= Bibliothek für Bildungsforschung
17) Weinheim 2000.

Toppe, Sabine: Die Erziehung zur guten Mutter. Medizinisch-pädagogische Anleitungen zur
Mutterschaft im 18. Jahrhundert. (= Beiträge zur Sozialgeschichte der Erziehung 1) Olden-
burg 1993.

Völpel, Annegret: Der Literarisierungsprozeß der Volksaufklärung des späten 18. und frühen
19. Jahrhunderts. Dargestellt anhand der Volksschriften von Schlosser, Rochow, Becker,
Salzmann und Hebel. Mit einer aktualisierten Bibliographie der Volksaufklärungsschrif-
ten. (= Europäische Hochschulschriften, Reihe I, Deutsche Sprache und Literatur 1568)
Frankfurt/Main et al 1996.

Weißensteiner, Johann: Pfarrer und Gesundheit – Aufgaben und Funktionen der Pfarrseel-
sorger im Dienste der Gesundheit zur Zeit des Josephinischen Staatskirchentums. In:
Aigner, Thomas; Horn, Sonia (eds.): Aspekte zur Geschichte von Kirche und Gesundheit
in Niederösterreich. Vorträge der gleichnamigen Tagung des Diözesanarchivs St. Pölten/
Historischer Arbeitskreis am 27. September 1997. (= Geschichtliche Beilagen zum St. Pölt-
ner Diözesanblatt 18; Beiträge zur Kirchengeschichte Niederösterreichs 1) St. Pölten 1997,
pp. 103–125.

Wild, Reiner: Die Vernunft der Väter. Zur Psychographie von Bürgerlichkeit und Aufklärung
in Deutschland am Beispiel ihrer Literatur für Kinder. (= Germanistische Abhandlungen
61) Stuttgart 1987.

Wimmer, Johannes: Gesundheit, Krankheit und Tod im Zeitalter der Aufklärung. Fallstudien
aus den habsburgischen Erbländern. (= Veröffentlichungen der Kommission für Neuere
Geschichte Österreichs 80) Wien; Köln 1991.

Winklern, Joh[ann] Baptist von: Biographische und litterärische Nachrichten von den Schrift-
stellern und Künstlern, welche in dem Herzogthume Steyermark geboren sind, und in,
oder außer demselben gelebt haben und noch leben. In alphabetischer Ordnung. Ein
Beytrag zur National-Litterärgeschichte Oesterreichs. Graz 1810.

'Not very happy and mixed with a lot of nervousness'. The priest as therapist in Catholic mental health care

Harry Oosterhuis

Introduction

Between 1958 and 1965, a Catholic Pastoral Centre in Amsterdam was specifically established to provide mental care to homosexuals. The Centre was part of a Catholic mental health organization and was staffed by several clergymen and psychiatrists. Its establishment arose directly from contacts that had evolved in the 1950s between the Amsterdam-based homosexual rights organization and a number of Catholic clergymen, psychiatrists, and psychologists who were open to new scientific insights into homosexuality. Board members of the Cultuur- en Ontspanningscentrum (COC) realized that they increasingly encountered Catholic homosexuals who were in moral conflict and felt a need for mental support. The director of the Amsterdam Catholic organization for mental health, psychiatrist C.J.B.J. Trimbos (1920–1988), listened to the homosexual movement's criticism that the Church showed too little understanding for concerns related to homosexuality. With the knowledge of the Dutch episcopate and in collaboration with the nationwide Catholic organization for mental health, Trimbos took the initiative to establish the Pastoral Centre, which on the basis of 'psycho-hygienic insights' was equipped to provide mental support to Catholic homosexuals. The Centre was set up as an experiment and the experiences gained by care providers had to serve as a basis to advise the Dutch bishops on 'the pastoral approach of Catholic homophiles'.[1]

The realization and practice of care provision of the Pastoral Centre – the subject of this article – must be seen against the backdrop of specific changes in the thinking about homosexuality within the Dutch Catholic community since the 1930s.[2] Despite the Church's official rejection of homosexuality as unnatural and sinful, some influential Catholic physicians and clergymen expressed alternative biomedical and psychological viewpoints. Differentiation was made between sinful homosexual acts that should be condemned and possibly prevented and a homosexual disposition which in itself could not be considered a sin and which had to be accepted as a deplorable, pathological fate. The possible biological and psychological causes of a homosexual dispo-

---

1   Regionale Instelling voor Ambulante Geestelijke Gezondheidszorg Amsterdam Oud-West, achtste/negende jaarverslag van de Katholieke Stichting voor Geestelijke Volksgezondheid voor Amsterdam en omgeving (1959/60), p. 19; Overing et al (1964), p. 11; Sleutjes (1980); Warmerdam/Koenders (1987), p. 299.
2   See Oosterhuis (1992).

sition were debated extensively among Catholic physicians, psychiatrists, and clergymen. In the 1930s and 1940s some doctors, often supported by priests, experimented with psychotherapy, chemical therapies, and even castration, but others were more cautious about the possibilities of curing a homosexual disposition. In the 1950s psychological explanations of homosexuality as a flaw, a neurotic disturbance of normal development in childhood and puberty, gained ground among Catholic psychiatrists.

In close connection with the differentiation between disposition and behaviour, two distinct categories emerged: 'true homosexuality' which was purportedly determined biologically or psychologically by an innate drive, and 'pseudo-homosexuality', which was seen as contingent 'perverse' behaviour of essentially 'normal' men and women. From the point of view of pastoral theology, these two forms of homosexuality had to be differentiated. As confessors and spiritual advisers, priests would have to take counsel with a physician before making a judgment on homosexual 'sinners'. Only in the case of pseudo-homosexuality was such behaviour to be treated as a mortal sin for which the offender was accountable. Although the concept of pseudo-homosexuality had been introduced by psychiatrists, it was mainly defined in moral terms. Moral judgment on 'true' homosexuals, however, should give way to a medical or psychiatric diagnosis. Clergymen and doctors were advised to cooperate closely: they should come to a common understanding and judgment of homosexuality. This served in fact as the Pastoral Centre's basic starting-point. It should be noted that its homosexual clients did not simply serve as passive objects of pastoral and psychiatric interference. In this paper I argue that new ways of dealing with homosexuality were not simply imposed on clients from above as the result of a clear-cut pastoral and medical strategy; rather, they came about by muddling through a process of interactions between clergymen, psychiatrists, and Catholic homosexuals.

The clients and their problems

In the seven years of its existence, the Pastoral Centre provided care to a total of 211 clients, of which 166 records are still available.[3] This material is unique in that it offers insight into the practice of pastoral care on which little documentation is available, partly due to the confidentiality of the confession. Apart from correspondence involving clients or third parties (relatives, friends, employers, parish priests and other care-providers), the records contain reports from priests and psychiatrists of the Pastoral Centre in which they sometimes quote or paraphrase comments from clients. The priests involved wrote the most elaborate notes. This can be explained on the basis of the nature and

---

3   The records of Pastoral Centre are numbered 1 to 211. In my references I have followed this
     numbering, thereby adding the formal role of the author of the notes and, between brackets,
     the year the client involved first came to the Centre.

structure of the care provision. Because the Pastoral Centre primarily catered for individuals with difficulties regarding religious concerns, the first person they would talk to was a clergyman. Based on one or more conversations, he would write a report for either the Centre's staff or a psychiatrist, if one was brought in for the client's treatment which only happened if a priest or client deemed it desirable. This also explains the absence of a psychiatric report in many records. The psychiatrists, in their turn, would sometimes refer a client back to one of the clergymen. The extent, accessibility, and level of information in the various text records vary considerably depending on the practical function they fulfilled, the length of treatment (ranging from one session to a dozen or more over several years), and the frequency of the care-provision contacts (ranging from once a week to once every six months). Most notes were made on the basis of the first talks the care providers conducted with clients to establish the nature of their difficulties.

It is hard to ascertain to what extent the records provide a representative image of the situation and daily life of Catholic homosexuals around 1960. The information in the texts is not only fragmentary, but also strongly coloured by selection, the retrospective gaze, and especially the interpretation of specific problems by clients and care providers alike. In this paper I am concerned in particular with the interpretations of those who requested and provided aid, as well as with the divergent and changing formulations they used to articulate problems around homosexuality and potentially solve them. I have read the data in the records as (constantly shifting) meaning constructions of the actors involved and my description of them involves a historical reading of their (changing) interpretations. If information in the records requires it, I will also pay attention to the social context.

The Pastoral Centre's clientele largely consisted of men. Only 10 of the 166 records are about women.[4] In terms of age, clients in their twenties were represented most strongly, followed by clients in their thirties and by teenagers. The number of clients over forty was quite small. That most clients were younger men can largely be explained by the fact that the discovery and awareness of homosexuality and the interrelated uncertainties frequently gave rise to the decision to seek help at the Pastoral Centre. The large number of men around thirty struggling with their identity and sexuality suggests that around 1960, on account of the influence of social pressure and the isolation in which many found themselves, individual coping often proved difficult and

---

4   One can only speculate about the reason for this limited number. Several records suggest that the male gender of the care providers could form an obstacle for women to call in the Pastoral Centre's help and that the care providers took lesbian women less seriously than homosexual men. Perhaps this was tied to the image of women as sexually passive, an image that was prominent in particular in Catholic circles. Regionale Instelling voor Ambulante Geestelijke Gezondheidszorg Amsterdam Oud-West, Pastoral Centre of the Katholieke Stichting voor Geestelijke Volksgezondheid voor Amsterdam en omgeving (hereafter PC), client 142 (1962); psychiatrist 40 (1960); psychiatrist 36 (1959); psychiatrist 58 (1960); psychiatrist 141 (1962).

potentially lasted quite some time. From their occupation and education it can be derived that most clients came from the lower and middle classes. Slightly less than half of those seeking help at the Pastoral Centre did so on their own initiative. A small majority sought help at the Centre on the advice of others (priests, friends, relatives and acquaintances, psychiatrists and family physicians, employers, lawyers and probation officers).

Although the Pastoral Centre was geared towards homosexuals with problems in the religious domain, the care providers also addressed other concerns. Aside from the inner struggle with homosexual desires, conflicts at work and clashes between parents and children were given ample attention. Other recurring difficulties pertained to homosexuality in marriage, prosecution by police and the law, as well as relational problems. If one client was helped by being reassured in one or several conversations (or, at least, he no longer showed up afterwards), another client might need sustained counselling or referral to more specialized care providing services. Inasmuch as the problems were unrelated to Catholicism, I will largely leave them unconsidered here: my argument concentrates on the relationship between religion and homosexuality. In fact, not just Catholics knocked at the Centre's door: Protestants, Jews, and those not belonging to any church made up slightly over ten percent of the clientele.

Most clients came to the Pastoral Centre because they struggled with inner conflicts and feelings of guilt. Many complained about being rejected by the Church or a lack of understanding among the clergy. Often, parish and other priests[5] who reproached homosexuals for being sinful, denied them absolution, or urged them to suppress their desires, merely fuelled their inner struggle. A few priests viewed marriage as a remedy and advised homosexual men to begin amorous relations with women, sometimes telling them they were actually bisexual. Some followed the advice, much to their regret. Other priests insisted on psychotherapy or referred homosexual men to a psychiatrist. Before going to the Pastoral Centre, nearly fifty clients had already been advised to seek psychiatric help. Their stories suggest that in the 1940s and 1950s medical involvement with homosexuality varied widely: ranging from advice to accept one's leanings and learn how to lead one's own life to the encouragement to pursue heterosexual contact and marriage; from psychoanalysis, which would mostly end prematurely because of the long duration or high cost, to (hardly successful) attempts at a cure with the help of medicines, hormone treatment, or carbonic and LSD treatment. Sometimes psychiatrists suggested castration as an option, but in most cases this was not pursued. Out of all the clients, two men were actually castrated.

Despite many complaints about the clerical approach, the records do not allow one to conclude that crude rejection and repressive measures were the

---

5   To prevent misunderstandings, in this and in the next three paragraphs, I refer to the way priests in general, *not* the Pastoral Centre's clerical counsellors, approached homosexuality.

order of the day in the Catholic Church. The records reveal that many priests showed restraint or even adopted a benevolent stance. Some of them approved of a homosexual friendship or would comfort a man, for instance, by saying that 'his homophile tendencies did not cause any serious evil'.[6] A young man said that his confessor, who knew about his homosexual relationship, did not commit himself, 'probably not to make [the client] worry needlessly'.[7] The privacy of the confession offered priests the possibility to speak 'with two mouths'. In public they had to condemn homosexuality as a sin, but in the confessional they could take a more flexible and tolerant stance. Not only was there a gap between official morality and pastoral care practice; the reactions among the clergy substantially differed: 'some confessors accept it, others don't,' as one of the clients commented.[8] Other priests, again, refused to discuss it, perhaps believing that keeping it under wraps was the best remedy.

It is striking that from a young age many men had had ample sexual experiences, sometimes with friars and priests. Catholic institutions such as single-gender boarding schools, seminaries, and monasteries in particular offered opportunities for homosexual contact.[9] Regular sexual contacts might also last for years without those involved viewing themselves as homosexual, even if some of them would have felt 'different' or sinful. Likewise, they might not even know the word 'homosexual'.[10] And if they were caught, the sanctions were generally limited, often involving punishments that were common for other more or less serious 'sins'. For example, one psychiatrist wrote about a young man who persistently took the initiative of establishing 'sexual contact [...] with a number of fellow-pupils' at a boarding school that occasionally he was punished by teachers to do one hour of mandatory study in his free time'.[11]

The unpredictability or contradictions in pastoral care were in fact a source of anxiety among Catholic homosexuals. Many did not quite know what was proper or not and they went to the Pastoral Centre with questions about the nature and implications of purported Catholic norms. Were they allowed to have a friend or live together with one?[12] Were they supposed to confess having homosexual contacts or could one 'follow one's own conscience'?[13] Their discontent pertained not exclusively to the Church's interference and sanctions but rather to the lack of clarity and the unwillingness of many priests to speak about homosexuality. Some announced they no longer wanted to hide their homosexuality within the Church – probably the most common conduct

6   PC, priest 76 (1960).
7   PC, priest 73 (1960).
8   PC, priest 15 (1958).
9   PC, priest 15 (1958); psychiatrist 24 (1958); priest 38 (1959); psychiatrist 202 (1964); priest 17 (1958); psychiatrist 127 (1962); psychiatrist 179 (1963).
10   PC, priest 37 (1959); psychiatrist 46 (1959); priest 23 (1958); priest 119 (1961); psychiatrist 134 (1962); psychiatrist 178 (1963); priest 182 (1963).
11   PC, psychiatrist 180 (1963).
12   PC, priest 30 (1959); priest 116 (1961).
13   PC, priest 137 (1962); client 105 (1959).

in the Catholic world – because they experienced this as hypocrisy, as 'dishonest' and 'insincere'.[14] As a young man complained: 'you can never really be yourself.'[15] Many took a critical stance, wanting the Church to show a 'different attitude' or 'much more understanding and openness'.[16] One of the clients wondered: 'Is it not the duty of the clergy to point out to people (and why not from the pulpit) that as Christians they should show charity towards homosexuals as well?' He felt that the Church 'greatly fell short' and was guilty of 'banishing the homophile minority'.[17] A teacher felt that clergymen voiced 'the most ridiculous things' about homosexuality and an office clerk argued 'that a possible demand of the Church not to have sexual contact with a friend is simply ludicrous, because this cannot be excluded from the "friendship"'.[18] Likewise, other clients had trouble 'sensing the sinfulness of sex' and did not see why they should feel 'sorry and moral regret'.[19]

If it is hardly surprising as such that Catholic homosexuals had a hard time with the Church, it is quite revealing how they expressed themselves about it. Their formulations make clear that a sizable number of clients refused to accept any clerical 'sermons'.[20] Apparently, hushing up, self-denial, and leading a double life were no longer taken for granted. Many statements found in the records suggest a certain degree of self-awareness and assertiveness. Catholic morality was experienced as bothersome, but at the same time most clients did not want to leave the Church. Numerous clients in fact came to the Pastoral Centre because somehow they felt a need, as a 45-year-old woman put it, 'to reconcile Christianity and homosexuality with each other'.[21] They wondered whether one could lead a 'responsible' life as a Catholic homosexual and whether there was 'room for homosexual people in the Church'?[22] Some men even wanted to become priests or monks (which was not always welcomed by the care providers because these homosexuals would thus 'escape' their own feelings).[23]

The requests for help reflect the dilemma faced by many clients. Their comments suggest a highly religious sense of guilt and loyalty to the Mother Church on the one hand, and increasing doubts about Catholic morality on the other. Only few actually complied with the Catholic commandment of sexual abstinence. Notably those who lived in Amsterdam or who regularly went there to seek pleasure struggled with the discrepancy between religious doctrine and their own sexual behaviour. By the late 1950s Amsterdam had a

---

14   PC, priest 58 (1960); priest 137 (1962); priest 184 (1963); psychiatrist 132 (1962); psychiatrist 208 (1965).
15   PC, psychiatrist 151 (1962).
16   PC, priest 116 (1961); priest 35 (1959).
17   PC, client 76 (1960).
18   PC, priest 18 (1958); priest 19 (1958).
19   PC, priest 32 (1959); priest 35 (1959); client 2 (1958).
20   PC, priest 72 (1960).
21   PC, client 184 (1963).
22   PC, priest 73 (1960); client 189 (1964); priest 121 (1961); psychiatrist 124 (1962).
23   PC, priest 72 (1960).

gay reputation already, as well as a tolerant climate, particularly compared to other parts of the country, notably the predominantly Catholic South, where homosexual rights organizations were still unthinkable.[24] Lots of men had moved to Amsterdam because of its urban anonymity and the opportunities of the then already existing homosexual subculture to meet 'likeminded people' and to engage in sexual contacts. The city allowed one, as some men noted, to lead a 'life of your own'.[25]

Quite a few clients, however, had mixed feelings about their new life in Amsterdam. The city not only offered the opportunity of freedom and the chance 'to build a new life'[26], but it also gave rise to uncertainty, doubts, and the fear of solitude and a gradual moral 'downfall'[27]. Having hasty and multiple sexual contacts triggered feelings of guilt and internal conflict.[28] One of the Pastoral Centre's priests characterized the homosexual life of a 26-year-old youth leader as 'not very happy and mixed with a lot of nervousness'.[29] Many clients were torn between the enticements of Amsterdam and their moral conscience. Inner conflict and mental tensions occurred in particular, it seems, in situations where one could escape the social control of family, neighbourhood, and the Church, while traditional Catholic norms and values – though subject to erosion – still had a solid footing. 'Wants to enjoy life while not getting trapped religiously', as one psychiatrist in one of his reports concisely summarized the dilemma experienced by many.[30]

To most clients, freedom was attractive and within reach. As their autonomy grew, the Church's rejection was increasingly seen as unjust while its morality was more and more experienced as restrictive. On the other hand, many Catholic homosexuals still felt too attached to the Catholic world to discard its views and certainties. They shied away from liberty and autonomy. These entailed, as one of them admitted, that 'you enter into an unknown life', or, as another one put it, that you 'had to live life' on your own.[31] On account of the 'forced loneliness', 'the spectre of having to remain alone', a lack of certainty, and a sense of insecurity, many clients tended to view a homosexual life as 'difficult' and 'meaningless'.[32] The seeds of the desire to 'be who you are'[33] were present, but for most clients it was hard to imagine how their life would take on meaning outside the given framework of the Church, marriage, family, and work. Apart from religion, the prospect of no marriage and family

24 Roodnat (1960), pp. 92–108; Duyves (1989).
25 PC, priest 21 (1958); client 148 (1962).
26 PC, priest 154 (1962).
27 PC, priest 122 (1962); psychiatrist 89 (1961).
28 PC, psychiatrist 52 (1960); priest 37 (1959); priest 64 (1960); psychiatrist 180 (1963); priest 35 (1959); priest 74 (1960); psychiatrist 151 (1962); priest 76 (1960); staff 18 (1958); priest 63 (1960); priest 137 (1962); psychiatrist 132 (1962).
29 PC, priest 182 (1963).
30 PC, psychiatrist 156 (1962).
31 PC, psychiatrist 123 (1962); psychiatrist 177 (1963).
32 PC, psychiatrist 44 (1959); psychiatrist 134 (1962); priest 37 (1959); psychiatrist 41 (1959).
33 PC, psychiatrist 130 (1962).

– which especially in the 1950s and 1960s counted as the essential basis for a full and happy life – was a source of great anxiety.

These particular problems of Catholic homosexuals were partly an effect of social changes in the 1950s. Growing prosperity and social mobility had gradually increased the overall freedom to choose and move around. Established boundaries of class, religion, and between the city and the country faded, and this caused the contradictions between social practice and the restrictive Catholic norms and values to grow. Numerous clients were torn between the constraints of religious tradition and the wider possibilities of everyday modern life.

The care providers: their difficulties and solutions

One of the main objectives of the Pastoral Centre was to keep Catholic homosexual men and women in the Church. The care providers realized that many of them might be disappointed by the Church, but that was not yet a reason, in their opinion, to turn away from it. Clients who expressed all too harsh criticism of the clergy were considered 'aggressive', 'bitter', 'hateful', and 'obstinate', or were attributed a 'crude mentality' and 'strong oppositional leanings'.[34] At the same time, in order to prevent apostasy among homosexuals, pastoral care providers would need to show more understanding for this 'group of fellow-believers at risk', as one psychiatrist put it.[35] In their striving to help homosexuals by teaching them, as one of the care providers put it, 'a livable morality and ethics within the dos and don'ts of our Church'[36], they had to adopt a cautious approach. This care was provided with the consent of the Dutch bishops and within the established Catholic order it was not possible openly to discuss its religious morality.

The records regularly refer to 'new insights' used by the priests of the Pastoral Centre to reassure their clients who suffered from moral anxiety and sense of guilt. What these new insights exactly amounted to is hard to distil from their divergent and sometimes contradictory advice. Still, it is clear that commonly the clerical counsellors did not have ready answers to their clients' moral questions. The new pastoral approach gradually evolved through the experience gained in practice. The priests and psychiatrists regularly consulted among themselves, referred clients to another priest, and, if needed, would ask for advice from the Centre's moral theologian. If in one case a counsellor would speak severely to his client, telling him that he sinned or should refrain from sexual contact, in another case he would show more restraint and tacitly allow it. Care providers might insist on control and sublimation, for instance by telling clients to concentrate on work, study, hobby, or religious ideals, but

---

34   PC, priest 18 (1959); priest 32 (1959); priest 38 (1959); psychiatrist 54 (1960).
35   PC, psychiatrist 49 (1959).
36   PC, psychiatrist 49 (1959).

in other instances they implicitly if not explicitly suggested that it was permitted, or they would react stoically when their clients confessed their sexual experiences.

Like their clients, the care providers wrestled with moral dilemmas. The contradictions and ambivalences found in many of their reports cannot only be explained with the improvisational nature of pastoral care; they are also tied to the individualizing and psychologizing approach they adopted. The priests tailored their advice to the divergent personal circumstances and drives of their clients. It was essential which meaning of homosexuality applied to them. Was there a homosexual disposition or was it rather a matter of certain homosexual behaviours? Did it involve a love relationship or 'random' contacts? Did sexual interaction take place, and if so, was it motivated by love, or exclusively by lust? Before judging morally, the priests first had to establish whether or not someone was 'really' homosexual. The least doubt was enough for referral to a psychiatrist, the expert who could establish, as one priest put it, whether someone had 'a justified homophile inclination'.[37]

Time and again, care providers had to decide on whether or not clients were in fact homosexual. Their outward appearance could offer some clues. Phrases such as 'this is a real homosexual, also looks like one (not to be touched with a ten-foot-pole)', 'seems to me – also in dress and appearance – typically 100% homosexual', and 'overdressed, swinging boy' are quite common, in particular in the psychiatric reports.[38] In the view of the care providers, men whose language and gestures left a feminine impression, who dressed unconventionally – especially tight pants and suede shoes were conspicuous – or who displayed more than usual attention to outer appearance were unmistakable 'homosexual types'. In women they would notice specific masculine features.

But more important than their outward look was what the clients said about their sexual experiences, fantasies, dreams, emotional life, and childhood. The care providers attached much meaning to feminine predilections in men and alleged masculine features in women. Men who said that, as children, they had played with dolls, knitted, embroidered, and sewn clothes, or had liked doing household chores, enjoyed dressing up, and had had an interest in fashion thus confirmed that they had 'always been different'.[39] In addition, both the priests and psychiatrists devoted much attention to the upbringing of the clients and their relationship with their parents. Dominant mothers and weak or absent fathers are ubiquitous in the reports, while excessive mother bonding, disturbed relationships with fathers, and failed mother and father identifications occur frequently. If a limited number of clients was raised in a 'normal' or 'pleasant' family, many suffered hard times when growing up as a result of a lack of parental love, a lack of a 'warm' family atmosphere, a

37 PC, priest 51 (1960).
38 PC, psychiatrist 49 (1959); psychiatrist 183 (1963); psychiatrist 54 (1960).
39 PC, psychiatrist 146 (1962).

bad marriage of the parents, a (too) rigid upbringing, or a lengthy stay at boarding schools.

With their development-psychology and psychoanalytical perspective, care providers distanced themselves from the views that prevailed in the Catholic world and that linked homosexual behaviour to moral degradation, contagion, or temptation. The frequent questions of the psychiatrists about diseases and disorders, notably sexual deviations, among relatives seem to suggest they considered homosexuality as hereditary and physically determined, but it is more likely that such questions were part of their medical routine, and therefore we should not attach too much meaning to them. By and large, their interpretive frame was psychological rather than medical. Although they viewed homosexuality as an 'abnormality', 'deviance', 'defect', or 'lack', this did not imply yet that it was a disease symptom. The frequent references to mental disorders – qualifications like 'neurotic', 'unbalanced', 'disintegrated', and 'psychopathic' recur in the records – referred not so much to homosexual leanings as such, but to how clients reacted to social rejection. As 'outcasts' and 'banished', they suffered from 'loneliness', 'isolation', 'fear', and 'meaninglessness'.[40] The care providers did not go as far as suggesting that social and religious norms were responsible for social exclusion, as some clients did. Rather the care providers shifted the attention from the actual pressure of the social environment, which was hard on homosexuals, towards their inner coping with it. Where a man complained that he 'was despised by the masses and driven out of his job', a priest wrote: 'He is more than *sensitive*, sort of collapses every now and then, *feels* he is an outcast.'[41] Another man who constantly 'clashed' with his immediate surroundings, according to the priest, clung too much to what others thought about him; he lacked self-confidence.[42] About a student a priest noted: 'He *experiences* his homosexuality as very complex, fear of being expelled from society.'[43] Others had problems, according to the care providers, because they '*felt* banished', 'let down and frustrated by everyone', or 'repressed in their social life' and 'inhibited'.[44] Such formulations reveal the extent to which the care providers reduced social conflicts to an individual's emotional reactions to such conflicts. Still, they also observed the difficult social position of homosexuals: they were not as much sinful or ill than pitiful and in need of help.

That the psychiatrists distanced themselves from the common medical approach to homosexuality also shows in their reservations regarding a possible cure. In this respect several clients were pleasantly surprised. One of them, as a psychiatrist notes, 'slowly loosens up once he finds out that I am not going to

---

40 PC, priest 5 (1958); priest 15 (1958); priest 17 (1958); priest 21 (1958); priest 26 (1958); priest 37 (1959); psychiatrist 38 (1959); priest 106 (1960).
41 PC, client and priest 5 (1958) [my italics], cf. priest 79 (1960).
42 PC, priest 79 (1960).
43 PC, priest 15 (1958) [my italics].
44 PC, psychiatrist 10 (1958); priest 21 (1958); psychiatrist 38 (1959) [my italics].

treat him'.[45] Although some clients were referred to other psychiatrists for psychotherapy, it cannot be deduced from the notes whether they were meant to be cured from their sexual inclinations or from the associated mental and nervous problems.[46] In general the psychiatrists did not act on the request of clients or their parents to cure them of their inclination. Most had to accept that their leaning was 'incurable'. The only option for them was 'self-acceptance'.[47]

Inasmuch as the records can serve as evidence, the collaboration between the Pastoral Centre's priests and psychiatrists did not cause friction. The priests were progressive clergymen who were positive about professional mental health care. Still, several different emphases are noticeable. The psychiatrists showed less clemency with clients who continued to worry because of their religion. Where the priests showed much patience and understanding regarding the 'spiritual need' and 'pitifulness' of clients, the psychiatrists would observe a lack of 'sense of reality' and 'balance', and they characterized some, as far as their religious experience was concerned, as 'woolly', 'vaguely idealistic', 'oversensitive', 'sentimental', 'unstable', 'weak', or even 'hysteric'.[48] Several records suggest that the priests would adjust their initial emphatic attitude after consultation with the psychiatrist, shifting their attention from the clients' inner conflicts to their presumed mental defects, which was not always to their advantage.

Calling on psychiatrists in pastoral care more or less served as a backing for the priests. Catholic moral theologians tended to consider homosexual dispositions as such not as sinful. A human being was not free to choose his inclination, they argued, and this is why people could not be held accountable for it. In Catholic moral theology free will was a necessary condition for committing sins. A psychiatric examination had to establish whether someone was a 'real', 'manifest', 'original' or 'innate' homosexual, who 'outside of one's own decision' had this inclination and really 'could not do otherwise'.[49] A careful examination of the motivations was necessary for a well-considered moral judgment. It was important for the care providers to clearly distinguish so-called pseudo-homosexual behaviour from homosexual proclivity. Men and women who engaged in same-sex sexual interaction (or who might do so), and who did so not on the basis of some inevitable inner urge, but as a result of other causes and motives – such as habituation, financial reasons (prostitution), or an environment in which the other gender was absent – had to reckon

---

45   PC, psychiatrist 202 (1964).
46   PC, psychiatrist 114 (1961); psychiatrist 124 (1962); psychiatrist 109 (1961); psychiatrist 190 (1964); psychiatrist 207 (1964); psychiatrist 112 (1961); psychiatrist 209 (1965); psychiatrist 210 (1965); psychiatrist 36 (1959); psychiatrist 40 (1959).
47   PC, priest 13 (1958); priest 18 (1958); priest 37 (1959); priest 64 (1960); priest 173 (1963).
48   PC, psychiatrist 5 (1958); psychiatrist 24 (1958); psychiatrist 58 (1960); psychiatrist 76 (1960); psychiatrist 100 (1961).
49   PC, priest 15 (1958); priest 28 (1958); priest 34 (1959); priest 35 (1959); priest 37 (1959); psychiatrist 132 (1962).

with warnings and reprimands. Because they were essentially heterosexual, they ought not to evade the 'responsibility of marriage'.[50] When, on the other hand, the psychiatric diagnosis indicated a homosexual disposition, priests could justify safeguarding homosexuality from being judged in terms of sin and guilt. A psychologically based disposition made homosexuals essentially 'different' from 'normal' people. As victims of an inescapable lot they were in a 'special situation' and therefore, as one of the priests wrote, it was 'impossible to apply to them [...] the objective moral rules of the Church'.[51]

Besides possible homosexual behaviour of 'normal' men, the promiscuity and anonymous sex of homosexuals greatly worried the priests, and constituted a major reason for urging clients to go to confession. Although care providers advised some to move to Amsterdam, they also warned in advance against 'the frequent perils'.[52] Irregular and multiple sexual contacts were not just sinful, the care providers felt, but also a sign of mental immaturity. 'Seems really homosexual; has a hard time; is infantile, immature [...] ; still has a long way to go [...] towards building a full life', as one priest judged a 29-year-old man, who admitted that 'in times of intense sexual excitement' he engaged in multiple sexual contacts, without feeling too guilty about it.[53] Quite a few homosexuals, according to the psychiatrists, had a 'polygamous' or 'promiscuous' inclination and suffered from relational problems, unsociability, and 'loneliness', or found 'no peace' because they had no 'ideals'.[54] One of the priests said he was struck by 'homosexual people having little future, merely clinging to the present'.[55] By urging them to give 'meaning' to their life 'in normal society', thus sublimating their drives, as it were, care providers believed they could curb the risk of moral degeneration.[56]

Sex and friendship

Such advice and admonishments were in line with traditional Catholic morality, which offered homosexuals hardly any other choice but abstinence. This is not the full story, however. Although care providers constantly pointed to the perils of homosexual lust, they hinted at the same time at the notion that abstinence as a demand was little realistic if not unhealthy. In their view it was in fact not quite normal for homosexuals to refrain from sexual interaction. One

---

50 PC, psychiatrist 124 (1962).
51 PC, priest 49 (1959).
52 PC, priest 110 (1961); psychiatrist 13 (1958); priest 25 (1958); priest 38 (1959); priest 74 (1960); priest 48 (1959); priest 38 (1959).
53 PC, priest 89 (1961).
54 PC, psychiatrist 163 (1963); psychiatrist 198 (1964); psychiatrist 151 (1962); psychiatrist 30 (1959); psychiatrist 38 (1959); priest 110 (1961); priest 35 (1959); psychiatrist 7 (1959).
55 PC, priest 114 (1961).
56 PC, psychiatrist 24 (1958); priest 108 (1961); priest 94 (1959); priest 74 (1960); psychiatrist 44 (1959); psychiatrist 176 (1963); priest 108 (1961).

priest wrote that a very devout man who claimed 'heavenly bliss to be more valuable to him [...] than any physical contact whatsoever' – a view that according to religious morality was perfectly laudable – took 'a rather odd stance on such people'.[57] Other clients who in response to detailed questions from care providers showed little sexual interest and experience were seen to be 'undeveloped' or 'immature'.[58] 'My personal impression is that sexually this boy is nowhere yet', as one priest noted about a 25-year-old young man who could not accept his homosexuality and rather wanted to marry than give way to his urges.[59] According to the care providers some clients showed an 'irrational' 'rejection' and 'disgust' toward sexual matters.[60] The forced suppression of emotions and desires in some Catholic milieus, so they observed, frequently led to 'insincere feelings of guilt', unhealthy inhibitions, neurotic disorders, and frustrations.[61] The notes of one psychiatrist about a 26-year-old nurse – raised in a rigid Catholic family and suffering from 'horrible feelings of guilt' – underline that the care providers were aware that Catholic morality sometimes brought about serious mental problems: 'Fear. A constant feeling of deadly sin [...] Always obsession. Confession: always remained silent about everything. [...] fear-neurotic-depression picture.'[62]

The care providers' notes often reveal the tension between the duty to suppress sexual inclinations, as dictated by the Church, and the advisability of recognizing and expressing them for the sake of mental health. Sexual desires had to find a way out to prevent neurotic repression. The awareness that the traditional restrictive morality was at odds with mental health was a major incentive for the care providers to interpret theological guidelines broadly. 'Helping people' was quite different from 'imposing objective moral rules', as one of the psychiatrists wrote to a parish priest who objected to what he saw as unacceptable advice by the Pastoral Centre.[63] Homosexuals should not suppress sexual needs, but regulate them in a 'responsible' manner. The most striking innovation in pastoral care provision was the positive view of steady relationships, and this catered for a strong need among Catholic homosexuals. Many claimed to find 'happiness', 'security', 'a footing', 'peace', or 'safety' in steady friendships.[64] Under special conditions, sexuality within a 'good friendship' was 'responsible' and 'meaningful', the priests concurred, not only to prevent random sexual contacts 'out of carnal lust', but also to contribute to

---

57 PC, priest 106 (1960).
58 PC, psychiatrist 170 (1963); psychiatrist 190 (1964).
59 PC, priest 143 (1962).
60 PC, priest 79 (1960); psychiatrist 8 (1958); psychiatrist 167 (1963); psychiatrist 46 (1959).
61 PC, psychiatrist 167 (1963); priest 129 (1962); priest 8 (1958); psychiatrist 10 (1959); psychiatrist 30 (1959); psychiatrist 130 (1962).
62 PC, psychiatrist 210 (1965).
63 PC, psychiatrist 49 (1959).
64 PC, priest 26 (1958); priest 37 (1959); priest 99 (1961); priest 102 (1961); psychiatrist 120 (1961); psychiatrist 122 (1962); priest 137 (1962); priest 24 (1958); priest 120 (1961); priest 35 (1959).

'personal development'.[65] Sexual interaction was 'not a matter of sin and guilt' when the relationship was based on 'love' and 'loyalty' as in a good marriage.[66] Through self-examination clients ought to find out whether they could meet this moral condition and they had to be willing to account for their motivations. For example, one of the priests advised a 35-year-old man with moral worries 'not to pursue [lust] for its own sake, but not to consider sexual contact in the context of sincere friendship as sinful either', if at least he showed to be prepared 'to continue to be responsible – and not to disguise what was improper'.[67]

In some cases, care providers left their clients in the dark on purpose about the moral acceptability of sexual interaction. After a priest reassured a 21-year-old woman by saying that the 'inclination' and 'friendship' were not sinful, he left the question of the sinfulness of sexual contact unanswered by advising her not to deal with it 'until the situation presented itself'.[68] A priest advised a man with religious problems – who was refused absolution by his parish priest because of his homosexuality and who did not dare to take Communion without confession – to 'find out for himself whether it was sinful to him'.[69] Similarly, a woman who, troubled by 'moral conflict', came to the Pastoral Centre asking whether it was permitted that she lived together with a female friend, received ambiguous advice. Not because cohabitation was sinful or immoral, but because the psychiatrist felt she wanted 'to pass the responsibility for her actions on to us'. He wrote to the priest: 'not to tell her whether or not it was permitted; she herself has to bear the responsibility for it.'[70] When it came to the moral judgment of sexual relations, ambiguous advice was hardly an exception, and this might pose a challenge to clients who were used to the Church's carefully defined dos and don'ts. Some will have been left with more doubt and uncertainty rather than with less. One man wrote, for example, that he was fobbed off 'with spiritual talk' and he criticized the priests for their lack of clarity.[71]

Still, it is possible to discover coherence and structure in the advice provided by the Pastoral Centre. With its emphasis on self-knowledge, self-motivation, and personal responsibility pastoral care clearly displayed features of psychotherapy. From their frequent evaluative remarks on the communicativeness and verbal powers of clients it shows that the care providers did not favour a passive, wait-and-see attitude. Those who articulated their concerns well and were willing and capable of speaking candidly about themselves,

65   PC, priest 99 (1961); priest 184 (1963); priest 73 (1960); priest 110 (1961); priest 74 (1960); priest 184 (1963).
66   PC, priest 3 (1958); psychiatrist 116 (1961); priest 189 (1964); priest 28 (1958); priest 25 (1958); priest 26 (1958).
67   PC, priest 70 (1960).
68   PC, priest 40 (1959).
69   PC, priest 102 (1961).
70   PC, psychiatrist 51 (1960).
71   PC, client 76 (1960).

their personal history, and their intimate (sexual) experiences, and who also showed a view of their own on the issue, had an advantage over those who were less articulate. An active attitude and an adequate description of the problems were seen as first steps toward their solution. Having your own opinion, even if it came with a certain 'general contemporary'[72] criticism of the Church, was appreciated, particularly if the client considered himself co-responsible for the solution of his problems. Where their formulations stood in the way of a solution, the care providers tried to get clients to view their difficulties in a different light by changing the problem definition.

Instead of offering clear moral guidelines, which some clients in fact wanted from the priests, the care providers pointed out the importance of an individual conscience and own judgment. They sought to make clear to clients that a 'livable morality' was not imposed from outside or above, but was based on inner conviction. Clients were continuously stimulated to engage in self-reflection and moral self-judgment. Many who suffered from an awareness of sin and feelings of guilt were advised to consult their own moral conscience and formulate a judgment on their own about what was and what was not responsible. A man who worried about hiding his sexual contact with a friend from his confessor would be told at the Pastoral Centre that only 'what is *experienced* as sin' belonged in the confessional box.[73] In other words, as the priest told others as well, your 'conscience defines the level of guiltiness', while another priest noted in a record that some feelings of guilt were not 'real'; one could feel guilty 'against one's better judgment'.[74] In the eyes of the care providers the problem of many clients was that they viewed the religious dos and don'ts as an absolute moral standard and experienced it as an obligation imposed from outside and above. As one priest wrote about a client who appeared to be a 'convinced and practising Catholic': 'awareness of sin without insight. Based on written and overheard principles [...] in the area [of] religion: no feeling [...] little energy and autonomy.'[75] The priest wrote about another young man who came to the Pastoral Centre looking for 'certainty': 'Guilt complex. [...] [T]oo strong "worry" – springing from notion of duty.'[76]

In the specific ways in which the care providers interpreted and rephrased their clients' problems, attention shifted from rejection on the part of the Church and the sinfulness of homosexuality towards the way religion was individually experienced. One client, who 'had no conviction but still attended mass', was, as the priest wrote, 'religious in a superficial way'.[77] And the man who, according to the priest, just wanted to be reassured that he still belonged to the Church but was 'not very outspoken', was characterized as 'primitive'

---

72 PC, priest 137 (1962).
73 PC, priest 137 (1962) [my italics].
74 PC, priest 99 (1961).
75 PC, priest 48 (1959).
76 PC, priest 23 (1958).
77 PC, priest 2 (1958).

and 'superficial'.[78] In response to a client who still had problems with confession after the priest had explained to him that the measure of guilt was determined by one's own moral conscience, one priest wrote: 'Still has a very formal point of view.'[79] About another client, whom he comforted by saying that homosexuality 'was not a sin to him', the priest noted that the man did not 'internalize' this advice.[80] Apart from frequent qualifications like 'superficial' and 'primitive', the care providers also used such terms as 'immature' and 'undeveloped' to indicate that many clients' religious sense was not based on inner conviction, but merely on formalities, convention, or coercion.[81] The priests believed that a lack of internalization could lead to a frenetic attitude that might not only cause mental harm, but that might also cause clients to abandon their sense of sin impulsively. Clients who 'simply' felt 'there was nothing wrong with' homosexuality, or who said, for instance, 'it was no sin actually because [their] friend held the same view', reasoned, according to the priest, in an 'oversimplified' and 'primitive' manner and showed a 'narrow-minded moral development' or a lack of 'self-analysis'.[82]

Significantly then, the care providers shifted the emphasis from fixed religious moral rules to personal conscience and individual responsibility. This shows that pastoral care was shaped by a redefinition of Catholic norms and values. With their ideas about a 'livable morality' and a personal, individual way of believing the care providers stressed general Christian-humanistic values such as 'love of one's fellow-men', 'solidarity', 'understanding', and 'openness'. Many religious problems, according to the care providers, resulted from a religious experience in which coercion, passive docility, conformism, and fear prevailed. Their interpretation of Catholicism implied not only that sexual morality became slightly less suffocating, but also that believers had to meet other and psychologically higher standards. Many Catholics, raised on the basis of authoritarian principles, were inclined to take a passive or wait-and-see attitude and showed too little personal autonomy or initiative in the view of the care providers.

The latter not only applied at a religious level, but also, for instance, to the ways in which parents and children dealt with each other. Repeatedly the care providers voiced criticism of 'traditional' families in which 'paternalistically minded' fathers and 'devout' mothers took too rigid a stance and children had no opportunity of speaking with them 'confidentially' and 'openly'.[83] On closer inspection, unyielding Catholic parents were found to be too rigid and too austere. As one priest noted disapprovingly about a client's parents, who, as he wrote, reflected the 'standard type of [a] closed family': 'Everything must

78   PC, priest 80 (1960).
79   PC, priest 99 (1961).
80   PC, priest 26 (1958).
81   PC, priest 2 (1958); priest 24 (1958); priest 48 (1959); priest 79 (1960); psychiatrist 89 (1961); priest 102 (1961); priest 189 (1964).
82   PC, priest 102 (1961); priest 77 (1960); priest 102 (1961); priest 79 (1960); priest 75 (1960).
83   PC, psychiatrist 132 (1962); psychiatrist 155 (1962).

be cared for in minute detail.'[84] Not only did the care providers try to foster a sense of understanding with parents for their homosexual son or daughter; they also urged them to resolve conflicts by talking about them, through negotiation and compromise. Often they showed understanding of homosexual youngsters who tried to escape the rigid paternalism at home; in some cases they even encouraged them to assert themselves. One of the priests has the following to say about a young man who told him that his parents never had had time for him because of their demanding business: 'He himself observes that he protested against his parents, who, as he claims, provided no support, no guidance. But he hastens to add that this [protest] was of course wrong; told him that I do not quite know yet whether it was wrong indeed. There is a spark of opposition in his attitude when he talks about his home situation in this context.'[85]

The individualized and internalized experience of religion that served as standard to the care providers, as well as the assertiveness they sometimes encouraged, required another personality structure than the one fostered by traditional and authoritarian Catholicism. To develop into an individual with a self-reliant and balanced 'personality'[86], one who accepted his homosexuality and managed to give meaning to it in a responsible way, 'maturity' was needed. Condemnation in terms of sin, guilt, and moral degradation were replaced by other moral qualifications that had psychological overtones, such as 'infantile', 'undeveloped', 'immature', 'unbalanced', and 'unstable'. Rather than the clients' salvation, their mental health and resilience were centre-stage. Where clients articulated their difficulties in religious terms, the care providers often used psychological criteria. Both the psychiatric diagnoses and the pastoral advice that aimed at introspection suggest an individualizing and psychologizing mode of interpretation. Catholic homosexuals should let themselves be led in their behaviour neither by fixed rules and norms, nor by random impulses and emotions; instead, they had to find the right balance between the two based on careful inner evaluation.

By adopting an individualizing and psychologizing approach the care providers, trying to adapt Catholicism to the demands of social changes, exercised 'soft' coercion as part of the effort to teach Catholic homosexuals to deal with the increased social liberty. Genuine moral behaviour could not be imposed from outside or above, but had to come from within. Invariably the care providers insisted on self-guidance and self-regulation. The emphasis thereby shifted from prohibiting homosexual acts to adding meaning to sexuality through relationship development. Acceptance and understanding went hand in hand with a new, more subtle form of control. Apart from offering solidarity and support, care providers were also concerned with keeping their clients within the Church. The promotion of lasting and monogamous rela-

84 PC, priest 67 (1959).
85 PC, priest 114 (1961).
86 PC, priest 74 (1960).

tionships among homosexuals served as a strategy to keep them from pursuing random contacts and sexual interaction in public meeting places. Despite their 'being different', they could become 'simply the same' by conforming to the same moral order as married heterosexuals.

To what extent this pastoral care in fact met the needs of its clients and whether they followed the advice given to them is difficult to establish on the basis of the Pastoral Centre's records. There were some clients who clearly had no use for such counselling and they resisted it, actively, by expressing their discontent, or passively, by no longer showing up after one or two conversations with the priests. The care proved hardly effective for homosexuals who had already turned their back on the church. Others interpreted the advice to weigh the issues based on their moral conscience as a license for choosing their own lifestyle, and others again continued to brood over religious dilemmas. Still, a large number of records suggest that quite often the conversations with clients eased their conscience and that many accepted the pastoral advice with relief. In their efforts to bring Catholicism in line with social developments the pastoral care providers in particular met homosexuals who wavered as a result of the growing gap between traditional Catholic relations and the new social opportunities. If the various social changes made it possible for Catholic homosexuals to increasingly struggle out of those conventional relations, freedom, they realized, also came with uncertainties and problems of meaning. Many found a more or less temporary support in the moral guidelines of the pastoral care providers.

Conclusion

Although the clientele of the Pastoral Centre did not amount to more than a few hundred individuals during its short-lived existence, the Centre's influence has been quite substantial. In the early 1960s the insights gained in the practice of care provision were disseminated at conferences, in several publications and by Trimbos, who regularly voiced his views before a wide audience on Catholic radio. In a roundabout way, psychiatrists and clergymen expounded that for the time being medical treatment of homosexuals offered little prospect of a cure while moral preaching failed to solve anything. It was more advisable to accept homosexual dispositions, alleviate feelings of guilt, appreciate 'homophile' friendships, and tolerate sexual contact in steady relationships. Thus for the first time it became publically known that Catholic experts no longer subscribed to the clerical condemnation of homosexual behaviour.[87] Only later, in the 1970s and 1980s, similar voices were heard in countries like Germany and Britain.

This turning point in the attitude regarding homosexuality did not remain limited to Dutch Catholic circles. From the late 1950s, a similar development

---

87   Overing et al (1964); Trimbos (1961); Trimbos (1962); Trimbos (1965).

occurred among Protestants.[88] Within a few years confessional mental health experts and clergymen managed to bring about a change in the Dutch moral climate. Although the Netherlands were still a highly Christian country, this change contributed to the launching of the homosexual emancipation process, geared as it was to (self-)acceptance and social integration. This effort on the part of clergymen and mental health experts was marked by an apologetic, concerned, and quite ethical tone, calling not only for the sense of responsibility of homosexuals themselves but also on the compassion and solidarity of the Dutch population. It was not about sin or disease, they argued, but about the regrettable social discrimination and mental suffering of a vulnerable minority. Not homosexuality, but discrimination was damaging for public mental health. This approach, which was based on psycho-hygienic expertise mixed with a sizable dose of Christian-humanist 'solidarity', strongly contributed to a public debate in which moral condemnation of homosexuals was more and more difficult to justify and was interpreted as ignorance and prejudice.

The changing Catholic attitudes toward homosexuality should not be explained simply as a process in which mental health standards superseded religion; there was in fact a more complex interplay between the development of professional mental health care and religious values. From the 1930s homosexuality had certainly been progressively considered as a medical or psychological problem in the Catholic community, but at the same time it did not lose its meaning as a moral and religious issue. In fact, as appears from the records of the Pastoral Centre and from developments in the 1960s and 1970s as well, Catholic as well as Protestant pastoral care for homosexuals gained ground and was intensified due to the growing Christian acceptance of bio-medical and psychological notions of homosexuality.[89] Mental health did not replace religion, but rather contributed to a moral reorientation and a new pattern of Christian values, stressing the importance of individual conscience and responsibility as well as affection and fidelity in emotional relationships. Individual well-being and social welfare were re-conceptualized not only in terms of mental health, but also of spiritual self-realization.

The psychiatrists and clergymen of the Pastoral Centre tried to help Catholic homosexuals to find a lifestyle that conformed to (modernized) religious values. Especially the vacillating role played by the clergymen in their judgments is noteworthy; as moral guides they used the strategies of social work and psychotherapy. This can be explained in the context of the more general development of Catholic mental health care from the 1940s until the 1970s. Although the influence of professionals increased, the impact of clergymen on mental health care was far from nullified. While some clergymen tended to oppose the rise of modern mental health care, because they saw it as intrusion in their monopoly of treating personal and spiritual problems, others partici-

88   Janse de Jonge et al (1961).
89   Brussaard et al (1977).

pated in it. In the ongoing dialogue between clergymen and mental health professionals the meaning of Christian values as well as the definition of the object of psychiatry was transformed.

In the discourse of the Catholic mental health care of the 1950s and 1960s some central conceptions of traditional Catholic moral theology, such as freedom of will and moral accountability, played a crucial part. However, these terms became increasingly detached from theological conceptions such as sinfulness, guilt, the inviolable soul, grace, salvation, and redemption, and they were increasingly related to psychological notions such as personal growth, character, maturity, and self-reliance. Until the 1950s the object of psychiatry used to be defined in terms that indicated a lack of freedom and moral responsibility in the Catholic world. It was associated with the non-spiritual, with the turbid pool of irrational passions and instincts, which had to be subdued for the sake of man's salvation. In the 1950s however, the concept of freedom was used by clergymen as well as professionals in such a manner that it could be related to mental health standards in a positive way. Freedom was no longer perceived as an eternal supernatural essence of human beings, but rather as an ensemble of psychological capabilities that could and should be developed through good education and, if necessary, through counselling and psychotherapy. Thus, inside the institutions of mental health care, Christian values were given another meaning, so that they were in line with psychological standards. Passive obedience to moral authority was no longer seen as a virtue, and religious experience was to be rooted in inner conviction and confidence. Mental health, defined as inner freedom, was to be valued now as a precondition for a more individualized faith. Therefore, the central problem was no longer the sinfulness of man, but rather the lack of inner freedom of individuals.

Against this background the judgment of homosexuality by clergymen and mental health professionals changed twice during the 1950s and 1960s. While in the 1930s and 1940s attention had focused on homosexual behaviour (of 'true' as well as 'pseudo'-homosexuals), which supposedly infringed on the theological norm of spiritual freedom, in the 1950s reference was increasingly made to the condition of the minority group of 'true' homosexuals, who presumably suffered from a lack of inner freedom in a psychological sense. Homosexuals could hardly be held responsible for committing sins, because they were considered to be 'immature' and because they suffered from a 'deficiency in mind and free will'. Around 1960, as exemplified by the records of the Pastoral Centre, the second transformation took place. It was prepared by certain developments in mental health care, especially the impact of modernist theology, phenomenological psychology, psychoanalysis, and the human relations movement. These stressed the importance of individual authenticity and stable, emotionally fulfilling relationships between individuals as a refuge from the impersonal utilitarianism and materialism of modern society and as the modern mode of achieving religious values in personal life. In this context an important change in the Catholic judgment of marriage and sexuality took place: sexuality should not only serve procreation, but should be a way to express affection in relationships.

This shift from procreation to emotional relationships set the stage for a new view on homosexuality. If in the 1950s lack of freedom was supposedly situated in the psyche of homosexuals, it was now increasingly perceived as a characteristic of their social condition: they suffered from being looked upon as different and inferior, from being isolated and lonely, and from leading a meaningless life. Homosexuals could be helped now, not by treating their orientation – that had to be accepted as a destiny – but by supporting them to realize freedom in their lives. By promoting a situational and personalized morality, the priests and psychiatrists of the Pastoral Centre encouraged homosexuals to shape their lives in authentic and responsible ways. They were encouraged to work against their isolation and loneliness as well as their 'irresponsible and compulsory' promiscuity by striving for stable, lasting friendships. They were expected to overcome their lack of inner freedom, so that they might take part in the same moral order as married heterosexuals.

This approach was typical for the fundamental social policy change of the emerging Dutch welfare state which bore a Christian-Democratic stamp. Whereas 'deviants' had been labelled abnormal, immoral, diseased, a-social, and deficient before the 1950s, when they had been excluded from the healthy and virtuous body of society, now the strategies of pastoral and social work as well as of mental health care aimed at social integration. Now deviants such as homosexuals were supposed to be able to take part in normal society by developing their inner freedom, integrating body and soul, reforming their lifestyle and normalizing their social interactions. The emancipation of Catholic homosexuals from traditional church authority did not necessarily mean that moral control of sexual attitudes and behaviour disappeared. This control changed from external coercion to internal self-constraint. The Christian sexual reform meant that suppression of sexuality by rigorous divine laws, in which procreation within marriage was the standard, was superseded by a more humanistic ethical code, which stressed the meaning of sexuality for individual well-being and personal relationships. Pastoral care thus confirmed the importance and charged nature of sexuality and also unintentionally contributed strongly to a consolidation of homosexual consciousness and identity.

Bibliography

Brussaard, Anne Jetzonius Reinou et al: Een mens hoeft niet alleen te blijven. Een evangelische visie op homofilie. Baarn 1977.

Duyves, Mattias: Sodom in Maccom. Homoseksualiteit in de stadscultuur. In: Hekma, Gert et al (eds.): Goed verkeerd. Een geschiedenis van homoseksuele mannen en lesbische vrouwen in Nederland. Amsterdam 1989, pp. 235–248.

Janse de Jonge, Adriaan Leendert et al: De homosexuele naaste. Baarn 1961.

Oosterhuis, Harry: Homoseksualiteit in katholiek Nederland: een sociale geschiedenis 1900–1970. Amsterdam 1992.

Overing, Adrianus Fredericus Cornelis et al: Homosexualiteit. (= Pastorale Cahiers 3) Hilver-
   sum; Antwerpen 1964.
Roodnat, Bas: Amsterdam is een beetje gek. Amsterdam 1960.
Sleutjes, Martien: Studiecentrum voor Speciële Sexuologie 1953–1958. In: Homologie 3
   (1980), pp. 12–15.
Trimbos, Cornelis Johannes Baptist Joseph: Gehuwd en ongehuwd. Hilversum 1961.
Trimbos, Cornelis Johannes Baptist Joseph: Homoseksualiteit. In: Tijdschrift voor Politie 9
   (1962), pp. 265–268.
Trimbos, Cornelis Johannes Baptist Joseph: Homoseksualiteit. In: Katholiek Artsenblad 6
   (1965), pp. 218–220.
Warmerdam, Hans; Koenders, Pieter: Cultuur en ontspanning. Het COC 1946–1966. Utrecht
   1987.

MEDIZIN, GESELLSCHAFT UND GESCHICHTE – BEIHEFTE

Herausgegeben von Robert Jütte.

Franz Steiner Verlag   ISSN 0941–5033

Klinik der Universität Tübingen zur Zeit
der Entstehung der Geriatrie 1880 bis 1914
2005. 277 S. mit 61 Tab. und 27 Diagr.
ISBN 978-3-515-08654-7

25. Sylvelyn Hähner-Rombach (Hg.)
„Ohne Wasser ist kein Heil"
Medizinische und kulturelle Aspekte
der Nutzung von Wasser
2005. 167 S., kt.
ISBN 978-3-515-08785-8

26. Heiner Fangerau / Karen Nolte (Hg.)
**„Moderne" Anstaltspsychiatrie
im 19. und 20. Jahrhundert**
Legitimation und Kritik
2006. 416 S., kt.
ISBN 978-3-515-08805-3

27. Martin Dinges (Hg.)
**Männlichkeit und Gesundheit
im historischen Wandel
ca. 1800 – ca. 2000**
2007. 398 S. mit 7 Abb., 22 Tab.
und 4 Diagr., kt.
ISBN 978-3-515-08920-3

28. Marion Maria Ruisinger
Patientenwege
Die Konsiliarkorrespondenz Lorenz
Heisters (1683–1758) in der Trew-
Sammlung Erlangen
2008. 308 S. mit 7 Abb. und 16 Diagr., kt.
ISBN 978-3-515-08806-0

29. Martin Dinges (Hg.)
**Krankheit in Briefen im deutschen
und französischen Sprachraum**
17.–21. Jahrhundert
2007. 267 S., kt.
ISBN 978-3-515-08949-4

30. Helen Bömelburg
Der Arzt und sein Modell
Porträtfotografien aus der deutschen
Psychiatrie 1880 bis 1933
2007. 239 S. mit 68 Abb. und 2 Diagr., kt.
ISBN 978-3-515-09096-8

31. Martin Krieger
Arme und Ärzte, Kranke und Kassen
Ländliche Gesundheitsversorgung und
kranke Arme in der südlichen Rheinprovinz
(1869 bis 1930)
2009. 452 S. mit 7 Abb., 16 Tab. und 5 Ktn.,
kt.
ISBN 978-3-515-09171-8

32. Sylvelyn Hähner-Rombach
Alltag in der Krankenpflege /

Everyday Nursing Life
Geschichte und Gegenwart /
Past and Present
2009. 309 S. mit 22 Tab., kt.
ISBN 978-3-515-09332-3

33. Nicole Schweig
Gesundheitsverhalten von Männern
Gesundheit und Krankheit in Briefen,
1800–1950
2009. 288 S. mit 4 Abb. und 8 Tab., kt.
ISBN 978-3-515-09362-0

34. Andreas Renner
**Russische Autokratie
und europäische Medizin**
Organisierter Wissenstransfer
im 18. Jahrhundert
2010. 373 S., kt.
ISBN 978-3-515-09640-9

35. Philipp Osten (Hg.)
Patientendokumente
Krankheit in Selbstzeugnissen
2010. 253 S. mit 3 Abb., kt.
ISBN 978-3-515-09717-8

36. Susanne Hoffmann
**Gesunder Alltag im
20. Jahrhundert?**
Geschlechterspezifische Diskurse und
gesundheitsrelevante Verhaltensstile
in deutschsprachigen Ländern
2010. 538 S. mit 7 Abb., kt.
ISBN 978-3-515-09681-2

37. Marion Baschin
**Wer lässt sich von einem
Homöopathen behandeln?**
Die Patienten des Clemens Maria Franz von
Bönninghausen (1785–1864)
2010. 495 S. mit 45 Abb., kt.
ISBN 978-3-515-09772-7

38. Ulrike Gaida
**Bildungskonzepte der
Krankenpflege in der
Weimarer Republik**
Die Schwesternschaft des Evangelischen
Diakonievereins e.V. Berlin-Zehlendorf
2011. 346 S. mit 12 Abb., kt.
ISBN 978-3-515-09783-3

39. Martin Dinges / Robert Jütte (Hg.)
**The transmission of health
practices (c. 1500 to 2000)**
2011. 190 S. mit 4 Abb. und 1 Tab., kt.
ISBN 978-3-515-09897-7